Journey to Wholeness feels like the comfort of a best friend gently steering you back to the path of remembering your "wholeness." It's a wonderful, reassuring guidebook to inner and outer transformation by someone who's been there!

—Deanna Minich, PhD, International Speaker,
Educator, and Author of *Whole Detox*

Journey to Wholeness uncovers the deeply-rooted connection between our thoughts and our physical health. This book is an invaluable resource for health coaches and anyone else interested in women's health.

—Sandra Scheinbaum, PhD, CEO,
Functional Medicine Coaching Academy

Journey to Wholeness offers raw, compassionate…insights that will ignite the change women scour the internet and bookshelves for. In addition to physical healing, this workbook offers valuable emotional healing…as Dr. Champion expertly weaves her personal journey into guiding you through yours—to a destination guaranteeing the life you dream of.

—Karen L. Roach, LCSW

Journey to Wholeness

Dave & Judy —
Thank you for
being amazing neighbors!
I will miss you both

Jennifer

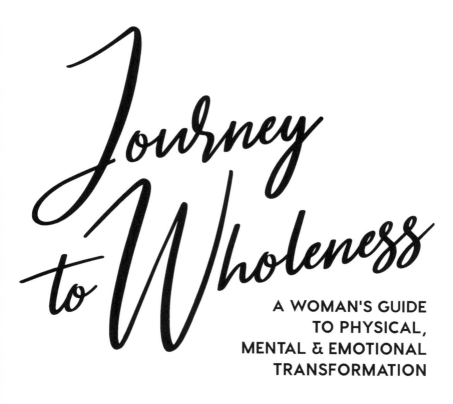

Journey to Wholeness

A WOMAN'S GUIDE TO PHYSICAL, MENTAL & EMOTIONAL TRANSFORMATION

Dr. Jennifer L. Champion

DCN, CNS, FMCHC, CN, HMCC

MEDICAL DISCLAIMER
The author of this book does not dispense medical advice or prescribe the use of any technique as a form of treatment for physical, emotional, or medical problems without the advice of a physician, either directly or indirectly. The intent of the author is only to offer information of a general nature to help you in your quest for health and well-being. If you use any of the information in this book for yourself, the author assumes no responsibility for your actions.

Cover design by MiblArt
Illustrations by Ruby Germany
Interior print design and layout by Michelle Nelson
Ebook design and layout by Marny K. Parkin

Published by NeoGenesis Nutrition, Inc.

ISBN 978-0-578-83054-4

THIS BOOK IS DEDICATED to the women who gave birth to me and who raised me, Michele Champion and Gayle Toohey, and to the women who have inspired me along the way.

To Tamra, thank you for loving me and encouraging me to get this book out of my computer and into the world where other women can take advantage of the journey.

You're not the same as you were before.
You were much more . . . "muchier."
You've lost your "**muchness**."

—Lewis Carroll, *Alice's Adventures in*
Wonderland & *Through the Looking-Glass*

Table of Contents

Acknowledgments

To my mother, Michele: Thank you for giving me life, even when it took yours. You are not forgotten.

To my grandmother, Gayle: Thank you for modeling what a strong woman is like and raising me to be one. I love you.

Tamra: Thank you for your unconditional love, unlimited support, encouragement, and editing skills.

Jaeden: You are such an inspiration and have made me a stronger woman and mother. If you hadn't taken the art classes, this book would never have been written.

Aurora: While you are a newcomer in my life, you help me see the world through a lens of color and creativity.

To my current clients: Thank you for bringing the challenging topics and your willingness to be vulnerable to our sessions. I continue to learn from you, as well as my journey. The depth of my gratitude for your trust is immeasurable.

To my future clients: You have the strength to work through the shadows of your past and live the kind of life you want. Believe in who you are and why someone put you here on this planet.

Preface

Grief, disappointment, and trauma are all etched into my own heart. I take solace that I am not alone in my experiences and that many women also experience these same patterns of growth in their own lives. From this shared experience came the concept for this journey book. This is no *read-and-put-away-for-a-rough-moment-later-in-life* kind of book. I have designed it to be fully interactive every step of the way. By allowing yourself to express yourself and live your life unafraid fully, you embrace the message behind this book. It is time to quit playing small and identify the triggers you have in your life that aren't just something of your past. Each of those experiences in the past gets lodged into your body and can create physical problems, symptoms, and diseases that no one wants.

I developed PCOS and lupus not because that was what my genetics told me I was going to have but because I buried my emotions, stuffed who I was, and tried to become anything that I wasn't. I filled my emptiness with food that wasn't good for me, activities that harmed me, and thoughts that reaffirmed that I wasn't worthy. Those negative emotions ate away at the normal functioning of my healthy body and created a body that

I loathed and wanted to throw away. I hated who I was and couldn't figure out why I was here on this planet. I wanted to find a six-foot hole in the ground and climb in—never to climb out again. But I didn't. I did not give up. I did not give in. You don't have to either.

Healing can be a daunting task. Vulnerability is a tremendous undertaking for many who have managed to bury emotions and hide their true selves deeply. Unearthing those skeletal emotions and events that have left us halted at one point or another in our lives can trigger a cascade of fear, anger, hurt, and sadness. However, like any dark period, we can count on the sun shining and the clouds clearing one day. No matter how much we have carried with us, we can put it behind us in a healthy manner— to put it down and not pick it up again because it's all we have ever known. All too often, the women in my practice share that they start on the right foot on the journey but soon find that they become fearful of the unknown. They know the abuse, struggles, and self-hatred. What they don't know is what is on the other side. Healing is a process and a journey in itself. Sometimes our travels are filled with valleys and peaks that impair our vision, and other times it's flat, and we can see for miles what lies ahead. It's in those times that we are unsure of what lies ahead that we learn to trust in ourselves and the learning we acquired from past experiences.

So, grab your favorite soft blanket, a cup of tea or hot cocoa, and a pen, and let's dive in. I am there with you as I so often longed to have someone there with me while I was doing the hard work. You are not alone. While my physical body isn't there, my heart is. My heart, my thoughts, and my energy are there with you in the form of this book. I am forever grateful that you invested in this book because it means you are investing in yourself, which brings me joy.

Introduction

My mother, Michele Champion, wanted me so much she married and reproduced with a man who had lost his way by succumbing to his history of abuse and anger. She died from systemic lupus erythematosus in 1983 at twenty-eight years old. I was five. Her mother, Gayle, raised me.

A powerhouse of a woman, my grandmother Gayle, worked her way up from a mailroom employee in a bank to one of its first female vice presidents. She pushed me hard to pursue education with my whole heart and mind, insisting I keep up my grades and find the courage to dig for answers. Because of her, my path led to my present life. I am forever grateful to her.

It has taken me years to accept what I just shared with you, and truthfully, it's sometimes still tricky. *My mother wanted me* and *I'm grateful for my grandmother pushing me* seem like simple, easy affirmations, but I've done a lot of hard work to reach a point where I can say them and mean what I say. My experiences on this journey have fostered my passion for helping others find their path to happiness. That's why I created this journal.

I'm going to ask you to dig into your story, past and present. You will face brutal truths and brave discomfort. Since I'll ask so much of you, it's only fair that I go first. I'd like to share my story with you.

After I lost my mother, I lived with my grandmother and step-grandfather. As mentioned, my grandmother was a powerhouse of a woman. I learned to push myself and never settle for just "good enough" from her. She was one of the first female vice presidents for a national bank when women didn't hold such power positions. That pressure, no doubt, drove her to drink. I remember many nights finding her passed out on the living room floor with the TV on and a glass and ashtray nearby. I have such compassion for her because I can imagine how she felt like she could never rest and always had to be outthinking and outperforming everyone around her. I still remember her telling me that if I wanted to get ahead in this world, I had to learn to be a bit androgynous—never conforming to what society told me was acceptable for a woman to do or be. Powerful words that have rung in my ears to this day. The downside of this mindset is that I learned that no matter what I did or how strong I was, it was never enough and that I would never be good enough. My step-grandfather valued animals above people, often treating the dogs in the house better than he treated me. He did not attempt to hide his resentment of me. He hated that he could not enjoy an early retirement because he had to take me in and would often fight with my grandmother over taking care of me while I was in the room with them. Raised among alcoholism and negativity, I heard things like "We had to work past our retirement to take care of you" "If you hadn't been born, your mother would still be here" and "She was a much better person than you are turning out to be."

I felt like I could do no right, please no one, and, indeed, shouldn't have been born. I understand now how those words often arose from stress and grief, but as a young child, I heard that my life was worthless, and I had no business being alive. Only while drunk did my step-grandfather ever express any positive emotion toward me. Otherwise, he never passed up an opportunity to remind me what a failure I was.

My family saw tears as a sign of weakness, so I trained myself as a child not to cry. As a sensitive and spiritual person, I found this difficult, but over time I learned to separate my heart from my mind. After all, thinking didn't hurt, but feeling sure did. I used this coping strategy to fight through two rapes, constant feelings of low self-worth, and years of emotional and mental abuse. I hated myself.

I tried to end my life in high school. Young me did not understand the error of burying my emotions, and I almost paid a terrible price. Fortunately, a friend and a volleyball coach caught me in time.

I so desperately needed to become whole, but I didn't know how. When it came time to start college, I wanted to move as far away as possible. I knew the stakes involved and felt the urgency to stand on my own two feet and find my voice. Even with such a high desire to change my life, it would still take me years to accomplish this goal.

Meanwhile, food served as a consistent comfort. Emotional eating champion right here! In fact, I took my emotional eating championship up to 350 pounds by the time I was a junior in my undergraduate program.

During my undergraduate years, I discovered I had a learning disability. I read at a fifth-grade pace, and quite frankly still do, but I learned to hide it because I didn't need any additional flaws. I didn't spend enough time reading as a child and spent far too many hours playing video games. Video games were something at which I excelled. It was a world where I could escape for hours and not have to listen to the negative comments made by children at school or family. In the world of video games, I was terrific. I was above reproach. All that aside, in college, I couldn't keep up with the reading assignments and felt like a failure. My inability to keep pace with my classmates forced me to change majors from journalism and English to psychology, and I fell in love with how the mind worked. Now, for some, obtaining a degree in psychology may seem like it would be far more tedious and academically rigorous, but for me, it was a comfortable fit. There wasn't as much reading, and there was far more observing behaviors and personalities. Observation and guarding were skills I mastered early on in life to survive. I didn't love school, but it came quickly for me and served as a place for me to hide. After graduation, I spent time job-hopping and not finding anything I loved.

In my early twenties, I was diagnosed with PCOS, or polycystic ovarian syndrome. My doctors put me on the three P's: prednisone, the pill (birth control), and Prozac. The prednisone made me gain more weight in a brief period, and I ceased to use it. The therapist prescribed Prozac because I was depressed—as are many women with PCOS—and the medical mindset of "crazy" rang in my ears as I filled that prescription. Eventually, I stopped taking Prozac because I didn't like the way it made me feel. The birth-control pills significantly increased my risk for gallstones and gallbladder disease, and I had to have my gallbladder surgically removed. Hormone-based contraceptives simply masked the underlying issues that create the right environment for PCOS to develop anyway, so it was better that I ceased using birth control. (Please note, this is not an encouragement for you to do the same. If you want to increase/decrease/cease medication usage, please consult your health-care provider before doing so.)

My mental and physical health issues, combined with watching my mother die from lupus, and my grandmother die after a series of strokes, inspired me to pursue studies in nutrition and health. Nutrition, exercise, meditation, correct supplementation (not just the latest and greatest advertised on TV or the internet), and the power of visualization helped me find the strength to make the necessary changes to get where I am on my journey. Each day I had to choose what foods I would put in my body and how I would move and think. It wasn't ever easy, but it did get more comfortable along the way as it became more routine for me. The same will happen for you.

This journey wasn't an easy one for me, and I certainly applaud you for taking the first steps on your journey. This journal is a reflection of some of the work I have done to feel more whole and a sample of what I use in practice with my clients on a daily basis. Every day that you get up, show up, and open up this book is a new day for you. It is a chance to focus on the positive and a chance to work toward becoming whole. What worked for me was to have the changes I needed and wanted to make to be broken down into tangible steps, pausing to ask, answer, and reflect on questions and ideas to which I had never given much thought. Then, from those thoughts, I was able to connect to my heart and focus on rejoining my mind and body. My desire for you is that you will one day be fully present and enjoying living life to the fullest every day.

Today, I enjoy getting up in the morning and checking my calendar. The opportunity to help each client makes all the blood, sweat, and tears of my education worth it! I also appreciate the opportunity to take control of my past negative experiences and direct them toward something positive. But I don't want to stop at only my clients. I want to use my experiences and education to help anyone who commits to working through this journal. If you'd like to become a client, no matter where you reside, you'll find my contact information in my author bio. I work with women who have hormone and autoimmune conditions, who come from all walks of life, and who can meet via phone and the internet.

Before you begin, here is a list of the supplies you will need on your journey:

1. A small journal, lined or unlined, preferably blank on the cover, but if you can't find one or you want to use one lying around your house, feel free to do so!

2. A large poster board. Any color is acceptable, but white may make things stand out more.

3. Magazines or online magazines/articles/websites that focus on appearance and our insecurities as women for their profit.

I hope you enjoy reading and working through this journal. Let it serve as an account of your journey. Turning the first page is like taking that first step. See you on the other side!

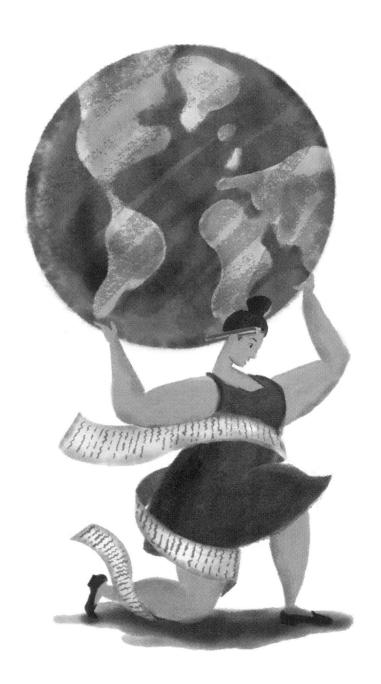

CHAPTER 1

Regaining Focus of What Matters Most

> *You change for two reasons: either you learn*
> *enough that you want to, or you've been hurt*
> *enough that you have to.*
>
> —Unknown

Section 1: Making Myself a Priority

1. I will accept that I am one person, and I do not have to do it all.
2. I will learn to say no. In fact, saying no is a good thing!
3. I will establish my boundaries and stick to them.
4. I will set small and large goals and celebrate my progress in healthy ways.

This first section focuses on accepting that you are *one* person. You cannot—literally and realistically—do it all. Yes, yes!

I know the pressure we face to do it all. From our makeup and clothing to our home lives and careers, the world expects us to at least look like we have everything together. Let's face it, though, ladies. That shit is HARD!

To achieve balance, we have to eliminate the things that do not move us toward our goals. While some of you already know what you want to accomplish, others are still trying to figure it out. Over the last couple of decades of my life, I've felt this overwhelming sense of being ridiculously and utterly behind. I'm not sure where this feeling comes from other than I fight with a tendency to judge myself by other people—a common thread that weaves women together. My friends graduated high school or college and then went off to be married and have families and maybe even successful careers. All the while, I felt like I was flapping and flailing my arms, trying to stay afloat upon life's ocean. What I have come to realize is that life comes to us when it is supposed to. No timeline matches another person's timeline. You are where you are supposed to be at this very moment in time. Even if you feel like you are lost or struggling, there are lessons to be learned that will benefit you later in this life and in the lives yet to be (for those who believe in reincarnation). It doesn't matter what age you are!

It is ok to have a career and no kids, a career and kids, or to be a stay-at-home mom and partner/wife. I've been in those categories, and because I now do the bulk of my work from home, I am both a career woman and a stay-at-home mom. No situation is easy, so let's cast aside any preconceived judgments we might have about "the other side" of womanhood. We're here to provide a support system for one another. We must stop buying into the idea of superiority and start learning from one another and building each other up. When we do this, we show up for one another and help each other achieve our goals.

The first step to building up the community of women is to start with yourself! Yes, *you*! A few years ago, on a show called *The Weakest Link*, the host would label the lowest-scoring contestant as the weakest link and then ask them to leave the stage. Throughout this journal, you will identify your weakest links—your old habits and unhealthy patterns—and ask them to leave.

To contribute to our community of women, we must let go of the things keeping us down. These can relate to our jobs, relationships, health, finances, spirituality, sexuality, internal conflicts, social outlets, etc. Anything keeping you from looking in the mirror and saying, "Damn, I'm fierce!" has got to go.

Weakest Links

Use the next few lines to write down anything that may be holding you back from achieving the life you want to live.

_____

_____

_____

_____

_____

_____

_____

_____

_____

_____

_____

_____

_____

_____

Now that you have written down the things holding you back, what will you do about them? Yes, I'm asking *you* what *you* want to do. Change starts with you!

Do any of these issues seem more manageable than others? Start with one or two of those. Even by working on the littlest things, *you will still make progress*. After all, every step forward has value, right? You are setting yourself up for success. In my practice, we focus on the path of least resistance or the smallest achievable goal. Sometimes it's exercising three times a week and for others, it's showering daily.

Let's go back to the idea of not having to do it all. Notice how I've asked you to pick only one or two things and not your whole list! You don't have to do it all right now!

When I started my weight-loss journey, I thought my entire life would fall into place. Guess what? It didn't. I felt like I had to clear the proverbial clutter from my life.

When I focused only on the physical aspect of losing weight, I lost less than when I included the mind-body element. So I decided to focus more on my lifestyle changes. I continued the physical actions of exercising and eating healthy, real foods, and I didn't berate myself while in the gym any longer. Instead of picking apart every little thing I felt was "wrong" with me, I allowed myself to focus on the positive steps I had made up until that moment and celebrate them no matter how small they might seem. I listened to my body when it was tired; I allowed myself to be done instead of pushing to do another set or lift a little heavier or run a little farther. I didn't run myself ragged physically, and yet I achieved better results. Why do you think this occurred? What is it about incorporating the whole person into the process of change that makes it more effective? Keep these questions in mind as you progress through your journey.

As we set goals and move into healthier ways of being, obstacles and naysayers will inevitably attempt to keep us from making these improvements. When others try to discourage you, stop and ask yourself what benefit they get from you staying in your present circumstance. I lost a few friends along my journey because as I made changes to better my health and my life, they had to take a hard look in the mirror, and it made them uncomfortable. Instead of joining me on what could be a difficult journey, it was easier to try holding me in my original position and maintain their comfort zones. This is **not** healthy. These are also **not** the people you need surrounding you. Friends should uplift and support you, encouraging you to be the best possible you. As hard as it may be, sometimes we have to reevaluate whether those we call friends deserve that title.

Family is a whole other issue. If you have a close, loving family, please reach out to them as they will most likely be your best support system. But what about family members who do not support you or, worse, actively try to discourage your efforts?

First, explain your point of view and gauge their reaction. Hopefully, it will be positive and you'll gain another supporter. However, if their response is negative, it's best to simply separate yourself from the situation and seek out a more supportive one elsewhere. Growing up, I had a difficult family situation and felt unwanted most of the time. It was much more effective and emotionally safe to reach out to those I knew would support me.

Look on the positive side! Who do you know that would support you? Who are your "ride or die" peeps? List them here with a couple of words next to each person's name as to why they made the cut.

_____

_____

_____

_____

_____

_____

_____

_____

_____

_____

_____

_____

_____

_____

A dream or a goal is more sacred than any possession, so you must protect it. This requires establishing and upholding boundaries. Do you find boundaries difficult? What usually happens when someone challenges your boundaries? Do you cave, or do you push back?

If you answered the former, it is time to strengthen your resolve. First, we must establish your boundaries. Look at the goals you have chosen to start with. Now, answer the following questions:

1. What are your boundaries? _____

_____

_____

_____

_____

_____

_____

_____

_____

_____

_____

_____

_____

2. What emotions arise when you think about the goal you
    have created? What feelings arise when you imagine
    accomplishing that goal? Keep in mind that the emotions you
    may be experiencing can be on both ends of the spectrum
    or somewhere near neutral. Try to avoid judging yourself
    for any of the feelings you might have. Right now you are
    to simply notice them.

_____

_____

_____

_____

_____

_____

_____

_____

_____

_____

_____

_____

_____

Now that you know your boundaries, you can directly respond when others challenge them. Yes, you may make some enemies, but at least the enemy will not be you!

Permit yourself to have setbacks and to grow from them. Setbacks happen, and no matter how minor or how significant, you can come back from them with new knowledge. Permit yourself to celebrate your successes. Even the smallest step forward deserves acknowledgment. Permit yourself to be your true self—the self who emerges when no one is watching!

Stop Carrying Your History with You!

One of my favorite movies is *Homeless to Harvard*. In the film, Liz Murray is a young girl raised by drug-addicted parents, who winds up homeless. Instead of giving up, she pulls herself up from the ditches and ends up receiving a full scholarship to Harvard University. Liz Murray's story and her final reflection as the movie closes gives me chills no matter how many times I watch it. At the very end, she looks directly into the eyes of the viewer and says, "I no longer have to carry my whole life with me. I can set it down."

In this section, I ask you to focus on setting down your past. Your past has shaped part of you, but it does not define you or your future. This section may require multiple visits to it for you to feel like you can fully let go. If that's the case, please know it's ok. No one's journey is exactly like the next person's.

For this next part, you will need a mirror. It can be any mirror where your hands can be free and you can clearly see your eyes. It best to see more of your body, so think big mirror!

Word of caution: I will be asking you to participate in breathwork in this next section. Practice this breathwork with caution, especially if you are new to it! For those unfamiliar with breathwork, there is a chance of hyperventilation if done too many times at too fast of a pace. To help prevent this, please take one or two regular breaths between the deep breaths of this next section. If you start to feel light-headed, please stop, rest for a few moments, and then move on to the next section. You can always return should you desire.

Stand in front of the mirror. Look deep into your eyes and concentrate. Is there is a scared, lonely, and hurting little one inside you? What did she experience? What are you holding on to for her? We all carry something—some part of our past that shaped us, molded us, and instructed us to hide parts of ourselves away because they were broken, bad, or wrong. Maybe you were older when this happened. Perhaps you didn't experience this type of pain as a young child, but you felt it in your teens. Maybe a parent or close family member died. Perhaps you had a tough breakup with your first love or had something very traumatic happen to you in your twenties. Time is irrelevant in this exercise as our inner child always lives within us. Once you have contacted her, recognize and hold space for the story she is telling you, then tell her she is loved and you will help heal her by establishing your boundaries and preventing anyone from hurting her.

Take a deep breath and release this breath with a whooshing sound. As you inhale, imagine inhaling all the things you desire in life. Maybe not all at once! We can't have you choking! What is it you want? The clearer you are on what you want, the more efficiently the Universe can bring it to you.

As you exhale, envision setting down whatever it is you are carrying with you. I like to think of myself having a backpack that carries various incidences of my past. I envision myself setting it down and walking away. Sometimes I mentally reach into the backpack and pull out a small item I associate with this moment in my past, and I put it in the trash. At times, I'm not ready to set the entire backpack down. Other times I am. Do what feels useful to you in this moment without judgment of self. As you set moments, items, or bags down, give the past one more hug before you let it go. Do this a second time if you wish, but too many times, and you may hyperventilate.

Without Our Past, Our Future Seems Less Glamorous

Embrace the present for what it is. An old platitude says the present is a gift, and it truly is. We have no idea what the future holds, and we cannot change the past. Changing the past would mean we would not be who we are today. Applaud yourself for the shit you have overcome, not because you deserved for it to have happened—you *definitely* didn't—but because you rose from the ashes. The anger and hurt you have carried around since that time is only hurting you, and your emotions can—and often will—affect you physically. And whether or not you see yourself as strong, amazing, and beautiful at this moment, you will see it one day as long as you are willing to shuffle your priorities a bit.

Make yourself your priority now. If you have kids, you can be a better mother to them by putting yourself first. If you have a significant other, you can become a better partner. If you are a CEO, you can become a better leader for your employees. When you become your priority, you create the space to be whole. It is a beautiful thing. The rest of the world will recognize all that you are and benefit from the example of your happiness.

I come from a long line of women who put themselves last. I learned it by default. It's not that they did it intentionally. It's merely what they learned from the mothers, aunts, sisters, grandmothers, etc., before them. They worked with what they had. Every night I would watch my grandmother run around the house like a crazy person trying to get everything done. She had the laundry, the cooking, the housekeeping, the work she brought home, and then there was me. There was never enough time to get it all done, and more often than not, I would find her passed out on the living room floor, in a drunken exhaustion. There was no time for herself. There was no time for her to take a bubble bath. No time to get a massage. No time to unwind and do something she loved. That is until her body made her stop. You see, the body will always find a way to slow us down when we are rushed and frantic.

The human body is not designed to continue at the pace with which we have become accustomed. Our bodies work a little and rest a lot more. Yet we find ourselves pushing our self-care to the back burner time and time again. Maybe it's a self-worth issue. Perhaps your anxiety is compelling you to always be on the move because if you stop, everything just might fall apart. Maybe you are trying to avoid the big emotions and feelings you have buried in you so deeply you are now afraid of what might happen if you let them out. Whatever your reason for pushing your own needs, wants, and desires to the back of your priority list, your body will catch up with you. The need for rest will overcome anything you have scheduled or planned.

One thing is true about this life. It is always changing and is, therefore, continually changing for you. I'm sure you realize what I am about to say here, but you get the opportunity to make the changes you want in your own life. *You* get to be the driver. *You* get to decide when you make a left turn or a complete

U-turn and create something new altogether. This includes prioritizing yourself and your own mental, physical, emotional, and spiritual health.

How do you do this? It's not easy in a society that wants to teach women we need to care for others. After all, for generations, we have been labeled as the nurturers or caretakers of the family. It's time we become the nurturers and caretakers of our own lives. It's time to prioritize yourself when confronted by the people, situations, or places that drain you. *Other people's rights and needs are not more important than yours.* If spending time with Aunt Susie emotionally or physically drains you, reschedule your visit. If going to a bar dredges up old, negative feelings about you or your friends, avoid those scenes. Say yes to the situations that bring you joy and fill you with happiness. Life is too short to always say yes to what we *don't* want and say no to what we *do* want because we think we don't deserve it. Try something new! Get out in nature and spend some time connecting with the Earth in a grounding and healing way. Try out that restaurant you've been eyeballing by taking yourself out on a date. Pick up that book you bought months ago and read it. What do *you* want to do?

I know that putting yourself first and rearranging your priorities can be a bit scary. Trust and believe in yourself. This may be the first time you have ever done this, but it is never too late to start! You have the tremendous power of intuition regarding your needs and abilities. However, society has urged you to distrust that intuition and seeks to define you and your capabilities. Only you should have that power, so don't give it away! Use your intuition, that small voice in the back of your mind or that feeling in the pit of your stomach, to help guide you. If you feel like you need help with your health, then reach out. If you feel like there are parts of your health you can address on your own or feel like you don't have the whole story, trust yourself.

Say no and mean it when you need (or just want) to! Say yes when you really want to and not just because you feel obligated. Human beings have used guilt to exert power over one another to the point we use guilt against ourselves. From where does the shame in your life come? Write it down, and then, below your story, please take a moment to write these words: "Guilt, you are no longer welcome."

_____

_____

_____

_____

_____

_____

_____

_____

_____

_____

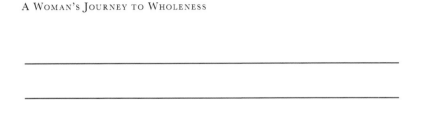

Section 2: You Aren't Atlas! Stop Carrying the Weight of the World on Your Shoulders!

Finding Balance in Life

I will accept that:

1. Doing it all is doing too much.

2. Perfection is a fraud.

I will identify:

3. The strengths I use in everyday life that help everything jive.

4. Areas on which I need to work.

5. Areas in which I'm doing well.

As women, we have learned to bear significant burdens. We have done so with our mouths shut and smiles on our faces for far too long. Day after day, we neglect our needs to fulfill the needs of others. Regularly carrying the burdens of others makes our bodies weary, our minds heavy, and our thoughts dreary. Enough is enough, ladies! We can only take so much. You do not have to hold the weight of the world on your shoulders. You were never meant to.

When we consistently overexert ourselves—mentally, emotionally, and physically—we create an overload of stress. This results in perpetual physical exhaustion. This is not all in our heads; it is our bodies crying out for rest and a safe place to unwind. When was the last time you answered your cry for help?

You see, the Women's Liberation movement ushered in our right to vote, own property, attend school, and hold positions we couldn't before. But it also ushered in extra stress. As we took on jobs outside the home, we were still expected to maintain everything within the home. Women are expected to bear children, return to work six weeks later, keep the house clean, further a demanding career, and do it while looking model perfect. Worse yet, we women tend to be our own worst critics. We look in the mirror and criticize ourselves instead of praising ourselves for all the things we do right. How many times have you crawled into bed only to have the tapes play all the conversations that didn't go the way you wanted, the things that were left undone from that day (or maybe days before because you still haven't had time), or berated yourself for not being good enough? Lay down the burden of judgment. It is tearing your health apart.

One of the topics I frequently explore with my female clients is perfectionism, or the idea that you must have it all, be it all, and never crack, break down, or show emotion. Perfectionism, ladies, is a complete fraud developed by our ancestors and passed down to us. Now, mind you, I am not blaming your mother or grandmother. The ancestors did the best they could with what they had—the same story they gave you. You, however, have the option to break this cycle of thinking perfection is necessary to be good enough. You are outstanding enough just as you are.

If there are areas you wish to change and *can* change, do it. If there are areas you want to change but *cannot* change (for example, your height), learn to accept it and love yourself, for there is no one else on this Earth exactly like you.

We all have strengths. Yes, even you! Exploring those strengths will help you determine your purpose on this planet.

What strengths do you have?

_____

_____

_____

_____

_____

How do you use them in your daily life?

_____

_____

_____

_____

_____

_____

Which strengths would you like to see increase in your life?

_____

_____

_____

_____

_____

_____

I was one of those women who thought I had nothing to offer. I even thought I would be dead by eighteen because I was so insignificant that no one would miss me. While other girls my age were planning for college and marriage, I remember sitting in my bedroom before my eighteenth birthday and writing out my directives. I had my entire funeral planned, right down to the type of flowers I wanted.

I was depressed. I was lonely. I was miserable. I bought into the ideology that I was not and never would be good enough. I heard the message of perfection everywhere, most frequently at home, but school was not far behind. On top of that, I beat myself down. If I succeeded at something, it was never due to any strengths I possessed. Nope! Just pure dumb luck that would be gone the next day. I wanted nothing more than to be as perfect as I perceived the other girls in my class.

Because I put that negative energy out to the Universe, it came bouncing back the next day, knocking me to my knees again. I did this day after day, not realizing I was punishing myself worse than anyone else ever could. I was punishing myself because I was unable to achieve an unreachable goal.

What goals have you created for yourself that you know are not reachable? For example, I used to want to weigh 98.6 pounds (I'm 5' 5") because I thought all of my problems would go away if I were skinny. I also pushed myself hard during my undergraduate years. I held three jobs, participated in theatre productions, held office in two clubs, and expected myself to get straight As. If I didn't, I was a complete failure.

_____

_____

_____

_____

_____

_____

_____

_____

_____

_____

_____

Ladies, stop dredging up past regrets. We all have moments in our past we wish we could do differently or that would produce a different outcome. That's part of being human. It's part of learning from the time we have here on this planet. Learn from your past and use that information to help guide and shape your future in a way that brings you joy, not more anger. You can use these moments to catapult you to a beautiful life. If you don't learn from them, they become a crutch, reinforcing the same negative thought patterns that created them in the first place. The choice is always yours: the crutch or the catapult.

Let's take a moment and break down some of the topics I just covered. We cannot know where to begin unless we start by telling our stories. I gave you a brief synopsis of mine, but this book is not about me. This book is about you traversing the path of healing from the inside out. Telling our stories gives us power over them. Choose one (false) idea or narrative you have adopted as your own. Write that story out. (If you feel a bit lost, you can return to the activity where you wrote about the things you think are holding you back.)

_____

_____

_____

_____

_____

_____

What did you notice about your narrative? Are there any underlying thoughts or tones in it?

_____

_____

_____

_____

_____

_____

_____

_____

_____

_____

_____

_____

Here is a trickier question. Through whose eyes did you tell your story? Wait! Before you answer that, go back and reread what you wrote.

Were the words you just read—your story—given to you by someone else? Can you hear the words rolling off your mother's or father's tongue? How about a former teacher? Pastor? Extended family member? Who told you this was the story of your life? Who told you who you would or could become? You see, we often haven't written the stories of our lives ourselves.

The blame game is not going to help at this point. Remember, what's done is done. The people in your past who contributed to the false stories you learned to believe were only working with what they had—their own misguided stories handed down to them from those who came before them. At this moment, you get to make a choice. Do you continue to live by the current narrative, or do you take the pen and start writing it yourself? You see, nothing is ever written in stone. We can change just about everything—except the past!

Look back at the narrative you wrote earlier in this book. What is something you wrote in your original narrative that you know isn't real? How far back does this narrative take you? Is it something you still believe? Is it something you adopted as truth when you were a child or a teenager? Use the next few spaces to rewrite those ideas. Transform them into who and what you want to become.

_____

_____

—————————————————————————

—————————————————————————

—————————————————————————

—————————————————————————

—————————————————————————

—————————————————————————

—————————————————————————

—————————————————————————

—————————————————————————

A journey of 1000 miles begins with a single step.

—Laozi

I once read this quote on a beautiful purple bookmark at a high school book fair. It resonated so deeply I have never forgotten it. That bookmark has lived inside some of my most treasured books and journals growing up. I never really had a space to express my thoughts or feelings in the living world, so I learned how to do that through the books I read and the words I wrote. I am still learning. Sometimes we don't get what we need from those around us, and we have to figure out how to find those things within us, no matter how deeply we have to search. For years, I buried all emotions. Much like many of the women I meet in my practice, I learned tears were signs of weakness and a distraction from getting things done. What I have since learned is that while tears can be an expression of pain, sadness, fear, and grief, they can also be expressions of joy, beauty, awe, appreciation, and amazement. While we can't always control the storms that produce the gray tears, we can revel in the moments we have the sunshine tears. Without knowing the pain, we can never honestly expect to envelop ourselves in the moments of joy and happiness.

Take a moment and reflect upon your achievements since you chose to put this book in your basket. Even a simple task, such as carrying this book to the register or clicking the checkout button online, is filled with conscious and subconscious decisions that have brought you to this point right now. You have chosen to do the work thus far. Maybe you have done some of it, or most of it, or perhaps you have done all of it. Wherever you are on this journey, this moment is worth celebrating. No one has forced you to do this work. No one has said, "You must do this or else!" Instead, you have reached this point of your own free will and choice. That is worthy of a celebration!

As I celebrate with you, I also want to keep the momentum going. Now that you are starting to see what direction you want to go, learning to utilize your strengths to make your next move can help. You may find it easy to identify your character strengths, or you may discover it to be a tricky, slippery slope.

If you have never thought you were good at anything or—dare I say—worth anything, let me reassure you. You have gifts, strengths, and worth. We *all* do! The fun part is recognizing these things as you transform your life.

Here is a fun and objective way to discover your strengths. First, ask your closest friend what strengths he or she sees in you.

What was his or her response?

_____

_____

_____

_____

_____

_____

We tend to be much harder on ourselves than others are, so don't skip this vital step.

Once you've done that, move on to the VIA Institute's Character Strengths survey, a great resource I use with my clients. Go to www.ViaCharacter.org and click on the Survey button. You can choose to purchase the reports if you would like more information on each of the strengths. However, you may simply right click on the free report and save it as a PDF for reference. Whatever you choose to do is perfectly fine.

What are your top five character strengths based on the VIA survey?

_____

_____

_____

_____

_____

_____

_____

_____

Reflect upon how accurate you think these results are.

_____

_____

_____

_____

_____

_____

_____

_____

_____

_____

_____

_____

_____

_____

_____

What surprised you most about your list of strengths?

_____

_____

_____

_____

Provide a few specific examples of where you use your strengths in daily life.

_____

_____

_____

_____

_____

_____

_____

_____

_____

_____

_____

_____

_____

_____

_____

_____

_____

_____

_____

_____

_____

_____

_____

Return to that same friend and share your results with him or her. What was his or her reaction? Did he or she see those characteristics in you?

_____

_____

_____

_____

Focus on Your Strengths Instead of Your Weaknesses

That Which We Feed Becomes Stronger

If you have experienced trauma, your perspective of life is probably different than others'. I am a survivor of trauma. My first rape occurred when I was in my early twenties. (It happened twice.) I know the anguish of feeling violated and how the fear that it could happen again seeps into the errands others run without a thought. I know all too well what it is like to wonder what I did to deserve this trauma.

I also know what it is like to feel abandoned, as my father walked out on my dying mother and me when I was five years old. I watched as my ailing mother weakened more and more until the day she died. Some thirty-seven years later, I still have the image of her in her hospital bed. I grew up without either of my parents, and while I had a family to grow up with, it was not the type of family my friends had. I felt ostracized and different when all I wanted was to belong.

Yes, I get what trauma is like. Mine may be similar or different from yours, but I'm reasonably certain our responses have not been that dissimilar. Do you know why I think this? Because you are still here reading the words I have written. I am certain a good deal of this book resonates with you! We are both survivors, which means we both have fighting, fiery personalities that have helped get us to this point. What matters most is not the trauma itself but our responses to what has happened.

Let's return to the idea of the crutch or the catapult. Which one did you choose? Are you using those past traumas as a crutch, or are you using them as a catapult? Though we cannot stop bad things from happening to us, we get to choose how we respond. How can you turn your trauma into something beautiful? In a moment, I will ask you to write down your trauma. Express it, put it on paper, give it life—and then I will ask you to take control of the life you gave it and stop allowing that trauma to have control over you.

You will make an agreement with yourself to stop punishing yourself for your past, for what has happened to you, for holding on to the anger and hurt that has consumed you. This can be any trauma—rape; molestation; the death of a child, parent, or other loved one; the loss of a job, the loss of a house, a miscarriage, etc. Write it here. Do not try to control your emotions while you are writing. If you are angry, be angry. If you are hurting or grieving, allow yourself to hurt or grieve.

_____

_____

_____

_____

_____

_____

_____

_____

_____

_____

_____

_____

_____

_____

_____

_____

_____

_____

_____

_____

_____

_____

_____

_____

_____

_____

_____

_____

Carrying these negative emotions destroys not only the human psyche but also the human body, and that is when we see dis-ease develop! It is time to let it go!

Letting-Go Activity

Put your hand over your heart. It's more in the chest's center behind the sternum (breastbone) and less to the left. I want you to focus on your heart. I want you to breathe into your heart. Concentrate on the smoothness of your breath as you inhale and exhale at a comfortable pace. Once you have brought your energy and awareness into your heart, allow the negative emotions you wrote about to arise. It's ok to cry. I'm giving you permission just in case you tell yourself that you can't cry or that tears are weak. Sit with those emotions. Recognize them. Thank them for being here and for the safety lessons they have taught you, and then let those emotions know they no longer are needed. When you say this to your negative emotions, I want you to also think of a positive feeling opposite to your original negative emotion. Imagine that positive emotion filtering into your heart as you continue to inhale and exhale. There are no "right" or "wrong" images or ideas for this new positive emotion. It can come to you in colors, thoughts, ideas, memories, etc. It is *your* positive emotion. Allow that positive emotion to fill your heart space, expressing gratitude for its presence in your life.

The Letting-Go activity can be done at anytime, anyplace. However, if you are driving while you are doing this, please, for the love of all things holy, do not close your eyes!

Learning to honor our emotions and hearts may be one of the hardest things a trauma survivor needs to learn to do.

Boundaries are often blurry for us. Trauma destroys boundaries. With this in mind, if you feel like you need a break from this work, that is ok. Maybe you need to rest and put the book down for a little bit. Take a nice deep breath—or perhaps even a long, hot bubble bath. Just remember to come back when you're ready. This journey is a marathon, not a sprint.

It is far too easy to focus on the negatives or the things we wish were different. As a society, we live for guilt. We are the only species that punishes itself repeatedly for the same mistake or trauma. We relive thoughts or moments in our heads over and over. We rehash topics with friends we know will commiserate with us but never actually give us anything to fill the positivity cup. We turn to drugs, alcohol, food, sex, shopping, gambling, and other reckless behaviors. We cope until we can't cope any longer, and then we melt. It's time we lived for something more positive!

I carried the negativity around for a long time, and I saw what it did to me. I sometimes still catch myself reverting to these thought patterns. In those small, dark moments, I remind myself how truly amazing, powerful, and fierce I am, and then I carry on with my day. I have learned to ignore the gremlins that lurked in my thoughts for nearly three decades. Now it is your turn!

Let's put those thoughts aside and focus on what we do well. Take a deep, cleansing breath: in through the nose and out through the mouth, making sure your exhalation is audible and longer than your inhalation. Close your eyes and imagine a large ball of bright, white light. Inhale that light in and allow it to fill you completely. This white light is here to heal you, to lift you and build you up as long as you will let it. As you exhale, imagine any darkness inside of you being pushed out and away from you. It no longer serves you, and so you do not need it. Let's begin!

What does this white light represent for you? What did the darkness mean?

_____

_____

_____

_____

_____

_____

_____

_____

_____

_____

_____

_____

_____

_____

_____

You completed some heavy work in this section. Return to it periodically. It may be easier to take one situation at a time.

Over the next few chapters, we will dive into our bodily systems and learn how our emotions and thought patterns can affect our physical health. But, for now, rest. Know you are loved, you are lovable, and you are enough.

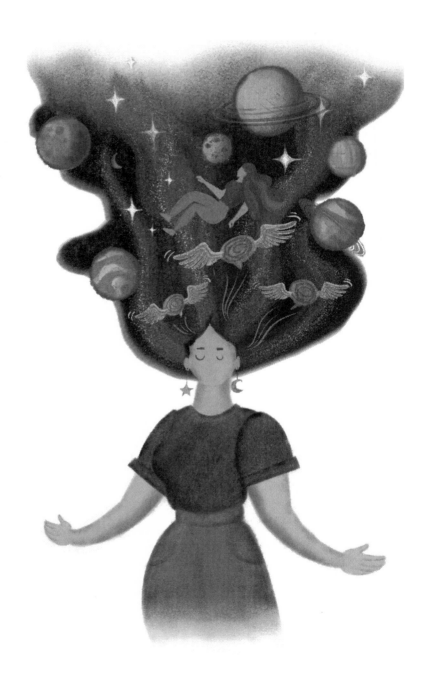

CHAPTER 2

My Thoughts, My Body, My Health

What We Think—We Believe—and
What We Believe—We Become.

Section 1: Creating Mindfulness

1. Just for today, I will not allow thought overload.
2. I can learn to develop a mindfulness practice.
3. I will take in the moments of awe and beauty.

Have you ever stopped and considered the thoughts passing through your mind? Probably not. We typically bumble along through our day, repeating the same processes from the day before and then press replay the next day.

To truly address some of the underlying issues such as trauma or physical symptoms that seem to have no explanation, we must learn *mindfulness*. In many cases, it is the missing link. Health practitioners have verified its value, making *mindfulness* a buzz-word. So, what is *mindfulness*, and how does one practice it?

Mindfulness is the art of being fully present in the moment. We don't look back at the past and conjure up regrets. We don't ruminate on the future and worry about what has yet to come. It is the "here and now" of our lives. We learn to savor the moments—the flavors, the smells, the laughter, the tears, the joy, the heartbreaks, the minutes that you will never get back.

Before we get started, be aware that practicing mindfulness can be challenging. Anything worth doing tends to be difficult, so always put forth your best effort.

Mind you, your best effort will feel different from day to day, and this is entirely acceptable. When life gets frustrating or disappointing, your best won't match up to the day, week, or month before.

Focus on the forward momentum of your efforts and try to remain positive. You **will** achieve your mindfulness goals.

Start the process of becoming more mindful by practicing breathing. Yes, breathing! Breathing helps calm anxiety, which in turn can improve overall health—without pharmaceuticals. It is also free!

As babies, we were naturally deep belly breathers. However, as time went on and stress weighed us down, we transitioned to shallow chest breathing. Our mindful breathing reconnects us to our original breath patterns.

You may feel light-headed while performing breathwork exercises, especially if you're not used to breathing like this, so take a seat or lie down. Listen to your body and make adjustments as needed.

One of my favorite breathing exercises, developed by Dr. Andrew Weil, is called the 4-7-8 breathing technique. YouTube has many demonstration videos, but the basic concept is to inhale for a count of 4, hold for 7, and then exhale for 8. It can take a few tries to find the right rhythm for you. For example, some of my clients report inhaling for an extra count because their lungs feel fuller.

Give it a try now. Repeat the 4-7-8 breathing pattern four times. Then record what you felt during and after the exercise. Notice any muscle tension, thoughts, etc. that seem to change from beginning to end.

_____

_____

_____

_____

_____

_____

_____

_____

_____

_____

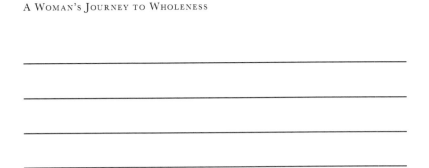

You can exercise mindfulness in many situations. As a clinical nutritionist, one of my favorite areas to practice mindfulness is around meals. People eat in their cars, on the run, and standing up while trying to feed others—none of which is healthy. We misinterpret internal cues and keep eating when we are full or reach for food when we are thirsty. We prioritize quickness and convenience over nutritious.

Why do we do this? Our society determines our worth as humans by how much we can get done in a day. Our meals have to fit our hectic schedules. It's a matter of survival, so we skip breakfast, drink coffee while we walk, and consider a homemade meal a luxury.

Another side effect of our punishing work ethic is that we tend to chew our foods partially. This puts extra stress on our digestive systems.

Healthy eating does not have to take a significant amount of time. Sitting for a two-minute breakfast of plain Greek yogurt (for those who can consume dairy) with raw honey and fresh fruit is far better than swallowing a jelly donut almost whole while racing out the door.

Which brings us to your next challenge!

Increasing mindfulness while eating can take awhile to master, so be patient. For the next week, pick one meal time during which you will emphasize mindfulness. Eat at a table without a television, computer, phone, or any other distraction. Of course, eating with others is a great way to build community and connection with one another, so feel free to enjoy or share a meal with friends or family. However, focus on only eating and nourishing your body without the digital distractions of today.

Savor each bite of food. What do you taste? Can you taste the seasonings? The food beneath the herbs? What is the texture and consistency? Have you chewed enough?

The first few times will seem awkward. I hear this often from my clients. It may even be downright uncomfortable at times. We multitask while we eat, and we have forgotten the pleasure and purpose of eating.

Use the space below to reflect on your experience of practicing mindfulness while eating. What was it like? What obstacles did you encounter, and how did you overcome them?

_____

_____

_____

_____

_____

_____

_____

_____

_____

_____

_____

_____

_____

_____

_____

_____

_____

_____

_____

_____

_____

_____

_____

_____

_____

_____

_____

_____

_____

Eating and breathing are essential, but mindfulness needs to penetrate all facets of your life. Start with your hobbies or interests. How can you be in the moment while engaging in these pleasant activities?

I started painting when I was about 15. (Let's not do the math here, please!) I have taken a few art classes, but nothing taught me the art of painting like mindfulness. When I made a vow to be fully present during my art moments, I realized how much more in tune I was with the brush strokes. My art flourished.

How much could you develop your interests if you practiced them mindfully, with no distractions? What would your experience be like? Are you brave enough to try it? Of course, you are!

Bravery & Mindfulness

I remember the first time I landed in Washington, USA. Trees lined the roads' sides, but the green "stuff" growing on the trees caught my eye. Growing up in the arid part of Southern

California, I'd spent the bulk of my life looking at brown: trees, bushes, grass, dirt, and sky. The sight of all that lush greenery awed me. I was almost shocked that a place like this existed.

My couple of days in Washington prompted me to put my house on the market. I had found my heart, my piece of beauty. I had no idea at the time, but one of the reasons I found my heart in Washington was my future wife. I just had to trust my intuition that this move was right for me.

Thirteen years ago, I gave birth to my son. I was amazed that this perfectly formed little being had come from inside me. His little head and his out-of-focus eyes were so precious. I simply could not imagine a more beautiful experience than holding that fleshy lump of perfection and calling him mine. How incredible!

Double rainbows, purple flowers, random acts of kindness—all inspiring moments that have brought tears to my eyes. Those tears are not weakness, but an involuntary expression of moments that take my breath away. What moments have taken your breath away? In what ways have they helped to shape who you are today?

_____

_____

_____

_____

_____

_____

_____

_____

_____

_____

_____

_____

_____

_____

_____

_____

_____

_____

_____

_____

_____

_____

_____

Section Two: Gratitude

Turning What You Have into Enough

1. Gratitude is an Attitude
2. Thirty Day Gratitude Challenge

Just for today, I will be grateful.
Just for today, I will focus on what I have.
Just for today, I will appreciate the little moments.
Just for today, I will love what I see in the mirror.
Just for today, I will not criticize myself but appreciate
    and recognize all that I have accomplished.
Just for today, I will love myself.
Just for today!

Remember the mindfulness activity at the beginning of this chapter? Well, here's a great place to practice it! Stop and take inventory of everything that is "right" in your world at this very moment. Stay in the present. For what do you have that you are grateful?

There are no correct or incorrect answers in this activity. Dig deeply and think about all the positive things you have going on.

_____

_____

_____

_____

_____

_____

_____

_____

_____

_____

_____

_____

_____

It is easy to get bogged down with negativity, focusing on what we do not have. I do not have a new car or a house. I am forty years old, haven't graduated from college yet, and I am overweight. I am so far in debt; I will never work my way out of it. Does any of this sound familiar? You are not alone in any of your sentiments. Millions of people share those same thoughts.

I have thought of many of the examples I listed, most recently the one about graduating. I felt like I'd been in school forever, but I happily concluded my educational journey with my Doctorate in Clinical Nutrition.

As the old saying goes, "Life is what we make of it." We can change much of the negativity we see in our lives, so long as we choose to focus on gratitude.

I am grateful for my education. Most importantly, though, I am thankful for the experiences and the personal growth I gained through the journey. Ok, I didn't have the choice in some situations as I *had* to take classes that I didn't want to, but I am still grateful! Whenever I've come out on the other side of a big challenge, I realized how capable and strong I was. That understanding is something to be grateful for all by itself!

Let's dig in and talk about ways that you can focus more on gratitude.

1. Stay in the moment—Sounds like mindfulness, right? Gratitude and mindfulness are intertwined. Researchers have found that those who practice mindfulness also have a greater sense of appreciation. What are you most grateful for in yourself and in your life? In what ways can you bring more gratitude to your focus daily?

_____

_____

_____

_____

_____

_____

_____

_____

_____

_____

_____

_____

_____

_____

2. For whom are you thankful? Write a thank you letter to that person. You do not have to give it to the person unless you wish to, but what better way to spread gratitude and smiles? Think about each word you put on paper and focus on the feelings this activity evokes. Grateful for your people? Say it! Remember, tomorrow is not promised, and thoughts are only useful if they are shared.

3. Speaking of which, when we smile, we release all sorts of positive, feel-good chemicals. They flood our brain and tell us everything is ok! A smile is also good for helping others feel better! Smiles are like yawns, contagious!

4. Break bread with people you care about! There is something magical about coming together with your friends and family

and sharing a meal. The laughter, the stories, the excellent food. There is nothing quite like it to lift your mood.

5. Go a whole day without complaining. Complaining is different than venting. You can have struggles, emotions, thoughts that you need to get off your chest. Do so! However, it becomes complaining if you keep doing it repeatedly while expecting to get a different reaction. We all have someone in our lives who complains about everything. Learning to find the joy in the situation will help you eventually let things go and move on to the more critical issues in life. Let's see how long you can go without complaining or focusing on what's "wrong" in your life. You can start small. Go a minute, ten minutes, an hour, a morning, etc., and work your way up to a day. Can you go even longer? Notice how it lifts your mood. When we forego a judgmental attitude, we become less likely to judge ourselves as quickly or sternly!

6. Take a walk and notice all the beauty around you. That should inspire gratitude! If it does not, why not? Do you live in an area that feeds your spirit or drains it?

7. Complete a Gratitude Journal—There is an activity in the next section below that can serve as a Gratitude and Service Journal for you. You may choose to use this next section, or you may decide to create a separate journal. Either is perfectly fine! If you decide to have an independent journal, I suggest selecting a blank-covered journal and decorate it. (Unless you are repurposing an old journal with a decorated cover) The decorating process helps build your mindfulness practice and also primes your mind to be open to gratitude.

Below you will find a 30-day challenge. You may choose to focus on that challenge exclusively for the next 30-days, or you may continue to work through this book concurrently. If you are working with me in a group setting, then I will guide you as to what to do during this time.

If you prefer a digital gratitude journal, several gratitude apps range from free to approximately $5.99. Find one that resonates with you.

Here is your 30-day challenge. In the following space, come up with at least five things each day for which you are grateful. Here is the trick, though—do not repeat anything during the 30 days!

Record your gratitude. It indeed can be anything! I've seen entries ranging from getting up in the morning to surviving cancer. When identifying 150 sources of appreciation over 30 days, you'll quickly discover how to look for and find gratitude in unexpected places.

For example, if I started my challenge on the first of the month, my first two entries might look something like this:

Day 1—Today, I am grateful for: the air in my lungs, the ground under my feet, being able to watch my son paint, having enough money to buy a meal for dinner, and the clothes on my back.

Day 2—Today, I am grateful for my cat, my house, my car, my intelligence, and my computer.

As you can see, it really can be anything- the only rule is that you cannot repeat any item over the next 30 days! Ready, set, go!!!!

Day 1 _____

_____

_____

_____

_____

_____

_____

_____

_____

_____

_____

_____

_____

_____

_____

_____

_____

Day 2 _____

_____

_____

_____

_____

_____

_____

_____

_____

_____

_____

_____

_____

_____

_____

_____

_____

Day 3 _____

_____

_____

_____

_____

_____

_____

_____

_____

_____

_____

_____

_____

_____

_____

_____

_____

_____

Day 4 _____

_____

_____

_____

_____

_____

_____

_____

_____

_____

_____

_____

_____

_____

_____

_____

_____

_____

_____

Day 5 _____

_____

_____

_____

_____

_____

_____

_____

_____

_____

_____

_____

_____

_____

_____

_____

_____

Day 6 _____

_____

_____

_____

_____

_____

_____

_____

_____

_____

_____

_____

_____

_____

_____

Day 7 _____

_____

_____

_____

_____

_____

_____

_____

_____

_____

_____

_____

_____

_____

_____

_____

_____

Day 8 _____

_____

_____

_____

_____

_____

_____

_____

_____

_____

_____

_____

_____

_____

_____

_____

_____

_____

Day 9 _____

_____

_____

_____

_____

_____

_____

_____

_____

_____

_____

_____

_____

_____

_____

_____

_____

_____

Day 10 _____

_____

_____

_____

_____

_____

_____

_____

_____

_____

_____

_____

_____

_____

_____

_____

Day 11 _____

_____

_____

_____

_____

_____

_____

_____

_____

_____

_____

_____

_____

_____

_____

_____

_____

Day 12 _____

_____

_____

_____

_____

_____

_____

_____

_____

_____

_____

_____

_____

_____

_____

_____

_____

_____

Day 13 _____

_____

_____

_____

_____

_____

_____

_____

_____

_____

_____

_____

_____

_____

_____

_____

_____

Day 14 _____

_____

_____

_____

_____

_____

_____

_____

_____

_____

_____

_____

_____

_____

_____

Day 15 _____

_____

_____

_____

_____

_____

_____

_____

_____

_____

_____

_____

_____

_____

_____

_____

_____

_____

_____

Day 16 _____

_____

_____

_____

_____

_____

_____

_____

_____

_____

_____

_____

_____

_____

_____

_____

_____

Day 17 _____

_____

_____

_____

_____

_____

_____

_____

_____

_____

_____

_____

_____

_____

_____

_____

Day 18 _____

_____

_____

_____

_____

_____

_____

_____

_____

_____

_____

_____

_____

_____

_____

_____

Day 19 _____

_____

_____

_____

_____

_____

_____

_____

_____

_____

_____

_____

_____

_____

_____

_____

_____

_____

Day 20 _____

_____

_____

_____

_____

_____

_____

_____

_____

_____

_____

_____

_____

_____

_____

_____

_____

Day 21 _____

_____
_____
_____
_____
_____
_____
_____
_____
_____
_____
_____
_____
_____
_____
_____
_____
_____
_____

Day 22 _____

_____

_____

_____

_____

_____

_____

_____

_____

_____

_____

_____

_____

_____

_____

_____

Day 23 _____

_____

_____

_____

_____

_____

_____

_____

_____

_____

_____

_____

_____

_____

_____

_____

Day 24 _____

_____

_____

_____

_____

_____

_____

_____

_____

_____

_____

_____

_____

_____

_____

_____

_____

Day 25 _____

_____

_____

_____

_____

_____

_____

_____

_____

_____

_____

_____

_____

_____

_____

_____

_____

_____

Day 26 _____

_____

_____

_____

_____

_____

_____

_____

_____

_____

_____

_____

_____

_____

_____

_____

_____

_____

Day 27 _____

_____

_____

_____

_____

_____

_____

_____

_____

_____

_____

_____

_____

_____

_____

_____

Day 28 _____

_____

_____

_____

_____

_____

_____

_____

_____

_____

_____

_____

_____

_____

_____

_____

_____

Day 29 _____

_____

_____

_____

_____

_____

_____

_____

_____

_____

_____

_____

_____

_____

_____

_____

_____

Day 30 _____

_____

_____

_____

_____

_____

_____

_____

_____

_____

_____

_____

_____

What was this process like for you?

_____

_____

_____

_____

_____

_____

_____

_____

_____

_____

_____

_____

_____

What did you learn about yourself?

_____

_____

_____

_____

_____

_____

_____

_____

_____

_____

_____

_____

_____

_____

What did you learn about those people to whom you gave?

_____

_____

_____

_____

_____

_____

_____

_____

_____

_____

_____

_____

_____

_____

Learning About the Past Can Help You Give to the Future

During my childhood, my grandmother told me about my mother saving her allowance to buy art supplies to make gifts for her friends. I inherited both her artsy side and her generosity. I truly enjoy giving to others. I am always on the lookout for things that can put a smile on my wife's or my friends' faces.

Have you noticed feeling better after giving of yourself? There's science behind this. Dopamine, serotonin, and oxytocin, the most common "happy" molecules, are part of why we laugh and smile. They flood our brains when we give to others and genuinely enjoy doing so.

Now that you have focused on what you are grateful for, we will change direction slightly and start looking at ways to give to others.

Let me reassure you that you do not have to buy anything at any time! You have something far more valuable than money—your time. You have the *time* to make one person smile each day. You might be saying, "Dr. Champion, I don't have time to sit to pee, let alone find the time to do something for someone else!" Well, we all have the same 24 hours in a day. Maybe you give something to your kids. Perhaps you give something to a coworker. These don't have to be people you randomly come across in a parking lot or something like that. Look around you! People surround you. Some of those people you may not even know the name of because you have been so busy trying to get that next promotion or to keep yourself from losing your shit with your kids! Happiness is addictive. Don't believe me? Let's try this! For the next 30 days, find someone who does not expect anything from you and give the gift of your time.

Want to continue to give to yourself? Find a way to give to another *and* be active! Consider walking your elderly neighbor's dog or helping a stay-at-home mom clean up her home so that she can rest or spend time with her kids. Compliment a woman whose outfit is just rockin' today! Truly listen and be fully present for a friend or coworker during a conversation. We don't necessarily think of these last two as giving a gift to someone, but they are. You have given a piece of yourself, of your time, to someone else. In a society that prides itself on always being on the move, you slowed down to say something nice or be there for someone else when she needed it most. Give it some thought and come back and journal about it.

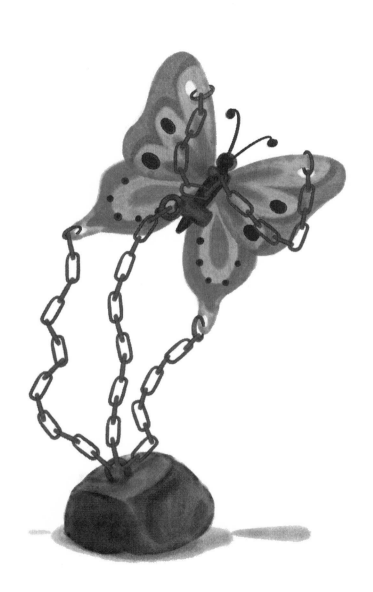

CHAPTER 3

You Are Good Enough!

*If you tell yourself something long enough,
you will start to believe it. How about
telling yourself the truth?*

Section 1: Vices and Change

1. I will no longer accept that I am broken. I am simply under repairs.
2. My vices are simply avoidance devices.
3. Change is inevitable and uncomfortable, but I am stronger and can do anything.

For years, I stuffed food in my mouth, hoping that it would numb the sadness and despair that lived within me. I grew up in a family that taught me that a facade was better than the truth.

I was raised by workaholic alcoholics, who focused on making sure that no one knew what was going on—in the family and within themselves. They self-medicated with work and alcohol, and I did it with food.

My mother passed away when I was 5. Although I did not fully understand what that meant in the long run for my emotional health, it stung later in life. Deep down inside, I knew that my family was doing the best that they could with what they had. They were reparenting at a point in life that they should have been enjoying their retirement and maybe even traveling. With me to raise, that retirement and travel remained elusive. They reminded me of that fact many times, but you know who else reminded me? ME! I carried around guilt and shame for who I was and why I was on the planet. I remember crying in my room and begging whoever was listening to exchange my life for my mother's. To bring her back and take me instead.

Food became my way of stuffing the feelings of guilt, shame, and abandonment. The worse I felt, the more I stuffed. And then, I felt guilty about the food that I ate because I was gaining weight, which became a focal point of my home discipline. The message I got was that I was only as worthy as the number on the scale. The higher the number on the scale, the lower my level of worth became. Eventually, food could not numb me enough, and I turned to alcohol.

I spent much of my early high school years in a buzzed state. I do not even recall most of my Freshman year. Sadly, the alcohol did nothing to help with the weight loss that I so desperately wanted to achieve. The weight loss, I believe, would have gained me acceptance from the people who were supposed to love me and protect me.

What are your vices? Are you a smoker that is trying to hide behind the stigma of "being cool?" Is the smoking habit a facade making it hard to see the real issues? Were you like me and chose food or alcohol? What are you trying to stuff down and drink away? Or are you on the other end of the spectrum and deny yourself nourishment because you feel unworthy or need to control some part of yourself that you don't like? Are you using your sexuality as a cover? Is sex or lust replacing love in your life? How about drug use?

It is even possible to have "healthy" vices that have gone to an unhealthy extreme, like over-exercising or restricting your diet to the point that you aren't getting all of the nutrients you need. Kind of like the good girl gone bad scenario! Are you taking healthy eating to an extreme that you can no longer enjoy your life? What are you trying to control?

Use the space below to tease out what your vices are. Be honest with yourself because you are the only person who is reading this. Acknowledge and be frank about what needs to change!

_____

_____

_____

_____

_____

_____

_____

_____

_____

_____

_____

_____

We all have a turning point. Make this one yours!

I remember back when I finally decided to lose weight. At my highest weight, I surpassed about 350 pounds. The scale was not able to register my weight at one point.

My PCOS (Polycystic Ovary Syndrome) symptoms were out of control. I was 28 and did not have a regular cycle, covered in excess hair and body fat. I was certainly not happy with the image that was staring back at me in the mirror.

I had tried everything to lose weight: diets, diet pills, exercise, starving myself, binging and purging—and nothing worked. Everything I did left me more discouraged and disappointed. At one point, I even considered suicide.

I lost my gallbladder and my sanity in the same summer. I remember lying in my hospital bed after the surgery and asking the doctor if any dietary changes could have prevented it or that I needed to change now that I lacked a gallbladder. He looked up from his clipboard and said, "Oh no, diet has nothing to do with the gallbladder. You don't need to change anything."

Let us take a moment to think about that! The gallbladder stores bile for the liver to help process fats in the diet. Mine was now gone, but I did not need to make any changes? Like the song from the 90s says, *"Things that make you go hmmm . . ."*

Even in my uneducated (at that time) brain, I *knew* that was not correct. It was at that moment that I knew I needed to make changes to my health. So, I did, and there was no turning back for me. I was tired of hating life and hating myself.

I was dating someone at the time who was following a particular diet plan (which will remain nameless because I do not agree with the approach anymore), and I picked up a copy of the book at the store and also joined a gym where I worked out six days a week. I followed it to the T, and I lost weight—105 pounds in fourteen months, to be exact. My cycle normalized, and I ended up conceiving my son.

Now I know you are asking yourself, "If she lost all that weight on that diet, why does she not like it?" It was a diet based on eating a lot of processed foods and foods with chemicals in them. Knowing what I know about the detoxification system and what can happen with an overload of chemicals, I choose to eat cleaner than the recommendations of that book I first picked up. Eating "clean" or eating whole, unprocessed foods focusing on vegetables, fruit, clean meats, and quality fats are critical for optimal health and wellness.

I hired a trainer to help me in the gym because I had no idea what to do and did not want to hurt myself! Even though I felt excitement, I did not lose my sensibilities! The trainer could only tell me how to use the machines safely and give me a workout routine. The rest was up to me.

It is up to **you** to make the necessary changes in **your** life. You can hire whomever you want to achieve your goals, but if you do not put in the work, then you will not get results. It is just that simple! As a doctor of clinical nutrition and functional medicine, I see clients with various goals. Just like no two snow-flakes are the same, neither are any two clients! However, the one thing that they all share in common is that they are *uncomfortable* with their current lifestyles. Without this sense of unease, they would not have come to me in the first place!

If you were comfortable with your life, your finances, your reflection in the mirror, your current lab values, you would not have purchased this journal because you are not ready to make changes. You are not in a position to put your full energy into making life better for yourself and potentially those around you. There is no judgment here. Where you are is where you are. Please put this journal down now and pick it up when you are ready to acknowledge your need and desire for change. It is ok not to be prepared, but I think that you are.

If you are still reading, this is where we pull out all the stops and get you going. If you are anything like I was a few years ago, you are sick and tired of being sick and tired. You have a whole list of things that you want to change, and you *are* ready!

Throughout the rest of the book, I will provide you with the questions to ask yourself and reflect on.

At this point in the journey, you are ready to fly. Scared? Good! Excited? Excellent! Those are good feelings to have in this instance.

I love to act, and one of the things that all of my acting coaches told me that if I do not have butterflies and nerves when I get ready to perform, I need to quit now. The same goes for making changes. The trick is learning how to keep self-doubt under your thumb and not above your head! It takes practice.

No one gets it right the first time. Hell! Even now after twenty years of working on my journey, I flub it up occasionally. It's what you do at that moment that defines your level of success. Give up or pick yourself up and keep trying?

We are continually changing and becoming better. I had an aunt once who told me that when we stop learning, we die. This death might be physical, but it is most undoubtedly mental/ emotional. The same is true of change. Once you feel like there is nothing else left for you to learn or change, then you have reached the end of your life.

You are not even close, sweetheart! So, get ready to buckle down and make something happen!

Section 2: Crutches and Catapults

1. Which instrument am I using?
2. Letting go is possible.

I remember when I met my son's father, and I asked him what he liked most about me at the time. He said that no matter what had happened to me, that I was not going to let my past hold me back from becoming the type of person I am to become. The same is still true today. Each day is a chance for me to improve what doesn't bring me joy and bring more color to what does!

All too often, we focus on the things in our lives that we are not doing "right" because we are still seeking approval from loved ones who did not give it to us earlier in life. But if we take a second and think about it, it is not about those people anymore.

The person we desperately seek approval from now is the reflection in the mirror. That is the only person who matters when the day ends. We have to go to bed with our consciences. We have to find a way to sleep at night with our choices.

I was very fortunate that I learned this lesson at an early age. Now, mind you, this does not mean that I don't struggle with wanting something more from the people around me from time to time. The reality, though, is that when I am living a life of genuine authenticity, I am much more at peace with myself—who I have become and who I *will* become.

I witnessed disease ravaging the lives of the ones who were on this planet to protect and to teach me. In a way, they taught me through their actions. You see, they were both alcoholics and overly stressed. I am sure that I was part of the reason for their additional stress, as they never intended to be raising another child in their later years, but I am *not* responsible for the choices that they made or the coping strategies that they chose. I am grateful for what I learned from them and many other adults who crossed my path. Without them, I would not be who I am today. What did you learn from those who raised you? Take a moment to brainstorm those things that you have learned and list them here:

_____

_____

_____

_____

_____

_____

_____

_____

_____

_____

_____

_____

Of those items on the list you just made, what are you still carrying around with you today? Or, as some might say, what is in the emotional baggage you are carrying with you daily?

_____

_____

_____

_____

_____

_____

The idea of the Crutch and the Catapult came to me one evening as I was conversing with my son's father. My response to the conversation where he said that I did not let my past hold me back was that I had to choose between letting the past be a crutch that would keep me crippled and immobilized or a catapult that would send me off into unknown greatness. Guess which one I chose? Every time someone told me no I said, "Watch me!" Every time I heard, "Not now." I said, "When?" Then I held them to that—or more importantly, I held myself to it.

If I was going to make it, I had to set an intention that I was not going to stop until I fulfilled the outcome of my decision. Not every decision was right! Trust me! I have my fair share of learning situations in my back pocket. Notice, though, that I did not call them mistakes or regrets. Life is not about amassing those—it is really about gathering all of the moments and situations that taught you something about yourself and the world around you.

The choice about how to view your history is always yours, of course.

Return to your list of those thoughts that you are still carrying around with you today. Are they serving as catapults for you or are they acting as crutches? Create two lists here and name them "crutch" or "catapult." Once you name the thought, it will be easier to decide if you wish to keep it or not.

Crutch	**Catapult**

Pick one of the crutches you wish to work on first. In the space below, describe what your life might look like if you turned the crutch into a catapult. What would be different? What feelings arise for you as you think about making these changes?

_____

_____

_____

_____

_____

_____

_____

_____

_____

_____

_____

_____

_____

_____

_____

_____

_____

_____

I can empathize with some of you on how complicated this process has been. I wish I could say it will all of a sudden go away. I cannot. I can, however, say that it will get easier. A habit becomes a habit (positive or negative) when you give it the love and attention it needs.

There is a parable I have heard often and has become my mantra over the years. It is attributed to the Cherokee nation. If that is true, I thank the people of that Tribe for this amazingly profound parable.

A grandfather is talking with his grandson and he says there are two wolves inside of us which are always at war with each other. One of them is a good wolf which represents things like kindness, bravery, and love. The other is a bad wolf, which which represents things like greed, hatred and fear. The grandson stops and thinks about it for a second then he looks up at his grandfather and says "Grandfather, which one wins?" The grandfather quietly replies, "The One you feed."

Food is a source of energy, and so are the words and thoughts we choose to have. They provide energy for whichever wolf we choose to care for inside of us.

I wish I could say that it is smooth sailing from this point, but I would be lying. This is where "shit hits the fan," so to speak.

Both of those wolves are very much alive inside of you right now. The "bad" wolf may even be stronger than the "good" wolf, but you can come to the "good" wolf's rescue. She has been waiting for your help, and now she can feel you coming to her.

Putting down the crutch and trusting that you will be able to walk to the catapult is monumental! Take a moment to acknowledge yourself for this! You may not have even seen the catapult until now, and that is all right. You may have been so reliant upon that crutch that you firmly affixed it to your body. It isn't. You *can* let go. The question is, do you *want* to? Are you willing?

There was a point in my life that my crutches were all that I knew. I could not see my way out of them. I was 13 when I first started drinking—a little bit here and a little bit there. Until one day, that *little* became *a lot*. I realized that alcohol had a blissfully numbing effect on me, and it helped me forget who I was—even if for just a little while. I allowed my drinking to consume me and carry me through to my Sophomore year of high school, where, sadly, I decided I no longer wanted to live anymore. I did not feel worthy of being on the planet and walking amongst my fellow human beings. One night, locked in my bedroom, I talked on the phone with a teammate from my high school volleyball team, and I told her what I was feeling—that I was tired and that I was going to kill myself. It was not a cry for help, not really. I knew where the alcohol was, and I knew where prescription pills were. I knew they did not mix. Enough of them, I figured, and I would sleep forever.

My teammate got on the phone with our coach, and the next thing I knew, the other phone was ringing in the house. My grandfather picked up the phone, and I nervously listened in the hallway. The end of the conversation I heard still rings in my head in my darkest hours, but instead, I choose to frame it in my mind as another one of my catapults. Sometimes we have to take a step back from our lives and ask ourselves what is real and what isn't.

I stood in the hallway and heard, "Oh, she does, does she? Well, let her go ahead and do it then. She won't be missed." Those words echoed in my head as I was whisked away to the local psychiatric ward for children. Those following three weeks for me—I will never forget. They gave me a chance to quit drinking and to start thinking. Considered a self-harm risk, I had all of my personal effects taken from me, and the therapist administered a battery of tests, including an IQ test.

My entire life, I had been told I was stupid, worthless, and that no one wanted me. While the latter two were still debatable, the first was no longer up for question. I was brilliant, and I had a test that *proved* it now. While some argue that IQ tests are unfair or illegitimate, what the test gave to me was light and hope. Those two things are immensely powerful in the process of healing.

Hope is both delicate and robust at the same moment. It can fuel some and elude others. Hope is the only emotion that I know can evoke confidence and fear in the same four letters. At that very moment, I mustered enough hope to be able to know I would be all right.

I no longer have to carry everything in my past with me. Neither do you. I am giving you some of my hope. Over the years, I have planted many hope seeds in my garden, and now I share them with you.

It is a seedling. It will require much attention and care on your part. The "bad" wolf loves to feed off of your fear and despair—it is all consuming. You must protect your seedling from the "bad" wolf. You must also be on the lookout for those who threaten to trample your hope seedling. Water it, give it food that will help it grow, and nurture it as you nurture yourself. If you do this, it will grow.

Take a look in the mirror. Now I want you to repeat the following words back to yourself:

"My life is full of hope. I am full of hope. I am rooted in hope."

Each day—for thirty days—I want you to repeat this to yourself every time you pass a mirror. At first, it will seem awkward and maybe a bit repetitive, but please give yourself the space to grow into these words, much like you are allowing your hope seedling to grow. It will become more natural over time. Also, snap a photo of yourself each day. Do not worry about looking "perfect" because unless you choose to show them to someone, you will be the only one to see these photos.

What do you notice about your face, eyes, and posture in the thirty days of photos and hope affirmation? (Come back here later to write about it.)

_____

_____

_____

_____

_____

_____

_____

_____

_____

_____

_____

_____

_____

Maybe you have been holding on to some negative thoughts about yourself. More than likely, those thoughts came from a time when you were still developing your narrative with the information you had. It is time to let go of those false ideas about who you were told you were. You have worked through rewriting and retelling the narrative of your life's story. You found places to be grateful when you thought there were none to be found. You identified areas you are ready to change and some that you are not. So far, so good! Look how amazingly strong you have been to even work this far along in the process. *You* have a lot to be proud of.

The idea behind this next section is derived from the field of positive psychology. Most counselors are trained to look at what is wrong in your life and how you can fix it. However, positive psychology looks at what you are doing "right" in your life and helps you apply your strengths (mentioned in a previous section) to the areas that you wish to change in the same manner as you do in the areas where things are working for you. For this chapter's final exercise, you will be examining the areas of your life where you are good enough. Don't worry! You have them. You have just been ignoring them while you focused on the areas in which you thought you were not good enough! Time to flip the script on your life.

Fill in the blanks:

I am good enough to _____

_____

_____.

I do a good job at _____

_____

_____.

I notice I really excel at _____

_____

_____.

I am good at _____

_____

_____.

I am good with _____

_____

_____.

I feel good when I _____

_____

_____.

I feel good when I am with _____

_____

_____.

I see the good in me when _____

_____

_____.

I amaze myself when _____

_____

_____.

I have a good time when I _____

_____

_____.

I Am Good Enough Because I Say I Am

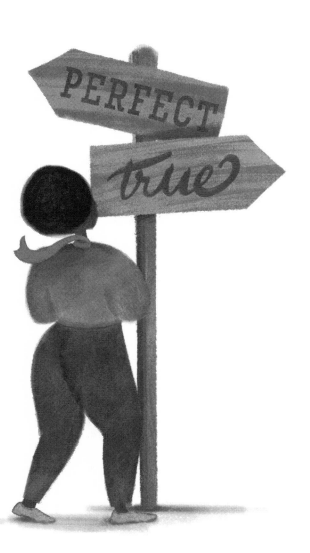

CHAPTER 4

Finding Your Self-Worth

> *No one can make you feel
> inferior without your consent.*
>
> —Eleanor Roosevelt

Section 1: Your Self-Worth is Not Determined by the Number of Followers You Have!

1. Stop editing your life
2. Let go of social media
3. Embrace life and the moments before you

Growing up, I remember looking at beautiful women and wishing I could be like them. I was very overweight as a child, which continued long into my adulthood. I would have given anything to be one of the beautiful girls at my school.

Beautiful is a relative term, is it not? We all have our beauty preferences. However, the media we consume heavily influences our society's ideas about what women should look, act, and be like.

With photo editing software, the media can take anyone, erase their perceived flaws, and make them impossibly attractive. A study conducted in November 2005 looked at the effects digital media has on self-image and perception. The findings surprised no one. The girls in Westernized society—that which included digital media—were more likely to have a decline in their self-esteem as they entered into their teen years (Clay, Vignoles, Dittmar, 2005).

Photoshopped celebrities creating an unattainable standard of beauty provides an ideal environment for marketers. Marketers want us to buy what they're selling. To do this, they convince us that we have to fix something—from our eyebrows to our waistlines—to be deemed worthy of existence. Our self-esteem takes a hit. What do you purchase to achieve worthiness?

Most of those images are not real. They present the illusion of perfection. Photoshopped alterations are only the final step to perfect an image that already includes professional hair and makeup, flattering lighting, custom clothes, layers of body-shaping undergarments, and an artist's eye. These images bombard us with the message that we should all aspire to that level of perfection at any cost.

Their marketing messages simply aren't true! *There is **nothing** wrong with you.* You are good enough the way you are, period. The perfect mish-mosh of your parents' DNA makes you unique. That is enough. You are not required to live up to artificial standards determined by editing programs and sales goals. If you wish to change something, do it! But do it for yourself and not because the media demanded the change.

When we feel unworthy, unattractive, or unlovable, we hide in the shadows. Holding back from the world does not contribute positivity and beauty. We learn to hide not only from others, but we also hide from ourselves. We begin to doubt our greatness. The reasons that we are on this planet in this moment become obscured by thoughts of deflation followed by depression and anxiety. Worse yet, by not testing our limits, we may never discover how far we can go. The fear of success is just as prevalent as the fear of failure, and so we hide.

One of my favorite quotes is from Marianne Williamson. You may replace the word "God" with whatever deity/energy/belief you choose to follow.

Our deepest fear is not that we are inadequate. Our deepest fear is that we are powerful beyond measure. It is our light, not our darkness that most frightens us. We ask ourselves, 'Who am I to be brilliant, gorgeous, talented, fabulous?' Actually, who are you not to be? You are a child of God. Your playing small does not serve the world. There is nothing enlightened about shrinking so that other people won't feel insecure around you. We are all meant to shine, as children do. We were born to make manifest the glory of God that is within us. It's not just in some of us; it's in everyone. And as we let our own light shine, we unconsciously give other people permission to do the same. As we are liberated from our own fear, our presence automatically liberates others.

—Marianne Williamson,
*A Return to Love: Reflections on the
Principles of "A Course in Miracles"*

Photo editing does not affect who you are. It cannot add to what you already possess. Look within yourself for the love and acceptance that you deserve. Once you realize this love has been within you all along, you will recognize it more easily from others.

This next assignment is an oldie but a goodie: Affirmations! Maybe you have tried them, but don't worry if you haven't! Either way, get ready because we are going to take them one step further.

Grab that stack of magazines or find some clippings/articles online that you mentally beat yourself up with every time you flip through the pages. You will also need a few photos of yourself and a large poster board.

Flip through the magazines or scroll through the website, looking only at the words. Disregard those images and move on. Even those models don't look like that. Cut out (or print) words that describe your current reality or your desired reality. What do you want to add to your life? What strengths do you want to develop further? These are the words you want to find.

Spread the photos of yourself around the poster board without gluing anything. Then match the magazine words to the images. What are the words and pictures telling you? What words did you find to match what you are feeling, thinking, or doing in the photos?

Using the words as category labels, start organizing your photos deliberately on the poster board. What do you notice? Take a moment to recognize what moved and why.

If you have a lot of open space, grab more photos and clip more words. Fill up as much space as you can. Once you have done this, affix the images and words to the board. You can use photo tape from the scrapbooking aisle to protect the photos.

This idea is a lot like Vision Boarding. However, most of the time, people create Vision Boards to imply forward movement in their lives. Your board focuses on the things that make you— **YOU!** You are not your career. You are not your hobbies. You are not your family. All of those things are part of you, but you are not those things. What do you bring to the workplace? To your hobby/hobby group? To your family? *Those characteristics make you who you are.*

You have now created a realistic picture of who you are. If you would like, you may extend this activity to become more in line with vision boarding by adding images or ideas of who you would genuinely like to become. If you choose to go this route, be careful to check in with yourself to make sure that these ideas aren't what society (or your family) *expects* you to become, but who you *truly* wish to become. Post this someplace where you will see it frequently throughout the day so it can serve as a gentle reminder of who you are.

We become used to seeing the images in the same place, so try moving the board from room to room. Alternatively, some of my clients like to focus on a different image each day, reminding themselves of their goals each time they look at it. Set yourself a goal. Take baby steps or leaps toward achieving it. You may also want to consider changing the photos around to focus on the ones that most closely support the goal you are working on at the moment. (You can use poster putty instead of glue for this since it allows you to move things around.) Find what works for you.

The next task will likely be more difficult, especially in our technology-driven world. The virtual world continually surrounds us. I'm connected to the internet as I type this and my phone is in my purse—also connected. However, our technology can become an addiction. Tech addicts check their phones, tablets, websites multiple times a day—some numbering in the hundreds of times. It is an obsession—and a psychologically dangerous one.

We humans have reduced our interactions to status updates and quick text messages, rarely communicating with one another in meaningful ways. Don't get me wrong; fast and convenient communication can be beneficial at times. For example, if I get stuck in a meeting that will make me late getting home, I can send a text to let my loved ones know not to worry. But how often do we use this technology for insignificant interactions like posting a picture of the dessert our waiter just delivered? Truthfully, no one cares what you are eating—well, except maybe me since I am a Nutritionist and Health Coach by profession.

I have watched the social media realm become a place to complain about things: ourselves, our environment, our neighbors! We complain about it all online. What does this accomplish? Not a damn thing! It makes us feel worse in the long run.

It takes away our power and gives it to the tech giant as we are intentionally shown images and ads that keep us scrolling. Your time is money and your psyche is how they control you.

When the complaint bank is empty, we post pictures, thoughts, words, etc. that is not our reality. It's the highlight reel for our lives. Social media is a facade, people! It is also primarily negative information entering your psyche. I'm sure you have heard the adage, *misery loves company.* Often, our social media posting supports this. I have posted cheerful or cutesy topics, educational articles and ideas, and posts about sadness, misery, grief, or doomsday. What posts do you think I receive the most interaction? If you guessed the last one, you are correct! Here's an example for you. I recently crossed the anniversary of my mother's death. She passed away on February 29, 1983. Leap year. I don't have to be reminded of this every year. Most of the time, I can move through February with a twinge of sadness but not the overwhelming grief. Not this year. Not 37 years after her death. It hit me like a ton of bricks. I picked fights with my wife, cried, and hid. I tried to escape in any way that I could. I wasn't willing to deal with this grief all weekend. That is, until I decided to post something on social media about it. I have about 1000 people on one of my pages. Out of those 1000 people, I had about 400 comments and reactions. On any other day, most people would skim through what I post, and maybe 10-15 people might react. Our society thrives on this type of interaction because it makes us feel like our lives aren't quite the shit-tastic circuses we believe they are. We look for confirmation that we are doing things right or that we're not as bad as the next person. We edit out the shameful moments and post only the prettiest moments, or we post attention-grabbing moments. What if we were just real with one another? What if we allowed ourselves to be vulnerable and know we are all connected in some way to one another? How might life change? Our society would change in many ways, allowing us to foster connections and communication that would feel fulfilling and supportive and not like we need to be an island.

Growing up, one of my favorite television shows was Dr. Quinn Medicine Woman. No surprise that I am now a part of the healthcare world! I loved how simple life was in those episodes. The characters made real food, ate meals together, and had a community. Yes, everyone knew everything about everyone, but before you cringe at the thought of your neighbors knowing intimate details about your life, isn't that what social media is? Human connection reigned in the mid-to-late-1800's. We were ourselves, not just a highlight real, but now the relationship is a lithium battery!

Here is your challenge. Delete the social media apps from your phone and avoid accessing them from your tablet or computer for at least a week. I hear you now! But this is how I stay in contact with so-and-so, or this is how I receive messages from my child's sports team or school. If there is another way to access this information or these people, try it out! If there is absolutely no other way, keep it to a once a day check-in and avoid scrolling to check out all of the other posts. Otherwise, cut off the bombardment of plastic, empty comments about how this is not right, that sucks, or FML—this pimple on prom night is catastrophic.

Over the week, journal about the experience. Start with the moment you realized I wanted you to delete your social media apps. What feelings did you encounter? If you felt stressed or anxious, how did you overcome those feelings? What did you notice about your moods and your connections with friends/ family over the week?

_____

_____

_____

_____

_____

_____

_____

_____

_____

_____

_____

_____

_____

_____

_____

_____

_____

_____

_____

_____

_____

_____

_____

_____

_____

Ready to go another week without those apps? How about a month? Once you take control of your time and focus, you create space to reconnect with those around you. Amazing things start to happen.

When we stop living digitally and start living authentically, we see ourselves in new ways. It becomes harder to compare ourselves to the altered and misleading images we see online.

You are good enough just as you are—at this very moment. There is no singular definition of perfection; it's all relative. What is perfect for you, the person next to you, or me isn't perfect for the next person. Which one of those matters? If you answered "perfect for you," then you guessed correctly. Remember this when you catch yourself judging yourself by anyone else's standards.

This isn't to say that society's standards are never worthwhile. On the contrary, they might, at times, help us improve ourselves. We need to be selective which ones we follow carefully. Are they attainable? Do they support my growth and well-being?

On the lines below, write one societally driven standard by which you tend to judge yourself.

_____

_____

_____

_____

_____

_____

_____

Is this an attainable goal? _____

If yes, what steps do you need to take to reach this goal? If not, then skip this section and let it go!

_____

_____

_____

_____

_____

_____

_____

_____

_____

_____

_____

_____

_____

Are these positive, healthy steps? Or are you depriving yourself of positivity and health to attain this goal?

_____

_____

_____

If they are not positive and healthy steps, is this goal attainable?

_____

Sometimes we have to take a hard look at what we have told ourselves that we want or need. We usually do not need these things. Do you need a larger house? That means a larger mortgage and more working hours to pay for it. Increased work hours take time away from our loved ones and other things we enjoy. Hmmm . . . well, that backfired! We do not need a luxury car. Yes, yes, I know! They are nice. They are well-designed. They carry prestige. But if you find that you must increase your work hours and decrease your quality of life, is it worth that misery? (Just a hint, if you are a sane human being, then you answered "no.")

What things do you truly need to be happy, loving, and thriving?

_____

_____

_____

_____

_____

_____

_____

_____

_____

_____

_____

_____

Now, let us get down and dirty and plan out how you will get those things. First tip: do not try to take on everything at once. It's hard to be successful when we're getting pulled in too many directions. That's when we start leaving projects uncompleted. Choose one or two of the things on the list and work on those first. Move on once you have achieved your initial goals. Look for items that would feed into one another. Can you prioritize your list in a way that makes sense?

Once you have picked one or two goals, fill this section out:

Goal 1: _____

What do I need to change to make this goal a reality?

_____

_____

_____

_____

_____

_____

What, if anything, do I need from those around me to make my goal a reality?

_____

_____

_____

_____

_____

_____

Who can I put on my team to make my goal a reality? What are their roles in this process?

_____

_____

_____

_____

_____

_____

Who and what does not serve me in this journey toward my goal?

_____

_____

_____

_____

_____

_____

What are my concerns about this journey?

_____

_____

_____

_____

_____

_____

What have I done in the past that enabled me to foster positive emotions and find my strength in the dark times?

_____

_____

_____

_____

_____

_____

_____

When will I know to call on my strengths on this journey?

_____

_____

_____

_____

_____

_____

Who can I contact when I feel scared or overwhelmed during this process?

_____

Who can I contact when things go well during this process?

_____

Where will I celebrate when I have reached my goal?

_____

Call that place and set the reservations for a specific date and time. Create a date or reservation to hold you accountable for achieving your goal.

Celebration date _____ time _____

Location _____

Dress to impress! You earned it!

Goal 2: _____

What do I need to change my thinking to make this goal a reality?

_____

_____

_____

_____

_____

_____

_____

What do I need from those around me to make my goal a reality?

_____

_____

_____

_____

_____

Who can I put on my team to make my goal a reality? What are their roles in this process?

_____

_____

_____

_____

_____

_____

_____

Who and what does not serve me in this journey toward this goal?

_____

_____

_____

_____

_____

_____

What are my concerns about this journey?

_____

_____

_____

_____

_____

_____

What have I done in the past that allowed me to foster positive emotions and find my strength in the dark times that I can apply specifically to this goal?

_____

_____

_____

_____

_____

_____

Who can I contact when I feel scared or overwhelmed during this process?

_____

Who can I contact when things go well during this process?

_____

Where will I celebrate when I have reached my goal?

_____

Call that place and set the reservations for a specific date and time. Create a date or reservation to hold you accountable for achieving your goal.

Celebration date _____ time _____

Location _____

Dress to impress! You earned it!

Repeat this process as often as you have goals to achieve. Your team must be a selective group that will support you. So, if you come from a dysfunctional family, do not recruit them for your team. If you are trying to avoid drugs, alcohol, gambling, sex, etc. then do not choose people who may tempt you to those behaviors.

What did you learn about yourself during this process?

_____

_____

_____

_____

_____

_____

What was the most eye-opening part of this journey? What did you learn from it?

_____

_____

_____

_____

_____

_____

_____

_____

_____

_____

_____

_____

_____

_____

_____

_____

_____

Section 2: Perfection isn't Real

Love Doesn't Demand That We are Perfect, Just that We are Willing to Accept Being Perfectly Imperfect

1. Perfection doesn't make YOU perfect.

2. The Path to Perfection is Titled "Crazy"

As I mentioned in the last section, perfect doesn't exist. Say it one more time because this is important. Perfect doesn't exist because what one person thinks is perfect isn't ideal for everyone else. We all define perfection based on our experiences, priorities, and values. These shape our personalities. The thing about perfection is that it drives us to become, or at least emulate, something we are not.

In my late teens, I wanted to weigh 98 pounds. I'm just under 5'5". In hindsight, I have come to understand why I saw thin as a standard of perfection.

I have always struggled with my weight. My family even used it to shame and punish me for my failures and mistakes. If I was late for school, received a bad grade, got into a fight with a friend, or anything else, my family blamed my weight. Therefore, if I was thinner, I learned to reason, none of these things would happen to me.

I didn't escape the torment at school either. Kids mocked me during PE, or as I sat alone during lunch and recess. I felt a need to isolate myself so that I wouldn't get hurt. Over time, I accepted that my weight was the source of my unhappiness. In turn, I adopted the belief that thinness equals perfection. The less I weighed, the better off I would be. For me, 98 pounds put me at a point I considered safe. If I were 98 pounds, I would not be fat. Society would not regard me as lazy or ugly. Maybe my family and "friends" would stop making fun of me.

I exercised for hours every day, and I ate as little as possible. Nothing worked, so I binged on the food I so desperately tried to avoid. This opened the door for guilt to nicely settle into my life. My skewed and dangerously unhealthy definition of perfection followed me for years. To be completely transparent, I still struggle at times with my few extra pounds. It is in those moments that I must remember to step away from the perfection gremlin.

I worked with a client recently, who shared her experiences regarding perfection. A tall, gorgeous, red-haired woman in her mid-20's, she had an olive complexion and sun-kissed freckles on her cheeks. She sat in my virtual office and shared the story she had carried for over a decade. Her mother and father fought a great deal while she was a young girl. They screamed at one another while she sat on her bed, rocking to soothe herself. The argument usually had to do with money scarcity, as she didn't grow up in affluent neighborhoods.

Flash forward to our current conversation. My client revealed that she never feels like she has enough money to cover the bills despite having a six-figure salary and a large savings account. She fidgeted in her seat, playing with a lock of her hair, and then looked up at me. She said she was tired of working so hard to chase the dollar. She wanted to have fun, but anytime she tried to take time off, she talked herself out of it for fear she hadn't saved up enough.

This young lady viewed perfection through a money lens. She perceived that she didn't have enough money to survive, so she lived in the pursuit of more money. She typically held multiple positions to ensure large paychecks. Through our work together, she learned to let go of her fears. We didn't focus on the money. That isn't the problem. Instead, we concentrated on the self-worth issues manifesting as her fear of lacking wealth. By recognizing when she was sabotaging her enjoyment of life, she started rewiring her brain and making new connections that worked in her favor. She eventually booked a trip to the Bahamas, where she relaxed on a beach with a couple of friends.

She realized her deeply rooted fears of financial insecurity were unintentional consequences of her parents' arguments over money. No matter how much she squirreled away, she would never have enough until she felt like *she* was enough. We assign no blame here. Her parents did the best they could with what their parents handed down, and so on through the generations. Instead of continuing the cycle, my client became aware of what she did and said that contributed to her financial fears.

Another client, let's call her Sally, felt obligated to take care of her mother even though her mother's negativity caused Sally's great distress. When her mother required more frequent care, Sally realized just how easily she became short-tempered. Her switch from a cheerful disposition to a negative one made her consider temporarily ceasing contact with her mother. She was exhausted. Her adrenal profile showed that the stress was causing issues and disrupting her sleep, sex drive, emotional stability, and hair loss. During one of our weekly calls, I asked Sally what she felt was best for her life at this moment. Through her tears, she said that she wanted to take a break from her mother, but her sense of daughterly obligation consumed her every thought. Her mother had seen her through childhood illnesses and hospitalizations; didn't that make Sally a failure as a daughter if she refused to take on the caretaker role now?

I asked Sally to paint a mental image of daughterly perfection. As she spoke, she revealed several areas where she felt like a failure, such as quality time spent with her mother. Instead of feeling fully present with the woman who raised her, Sally counted down the minutes until she could leave. She made lists in her head of everything she needed and wanted to get done. On many levels, Sally knew she wanted to make the most of the time left with her aging mother. She scolded herself for her actions but felt unable to choose differently.

It has taken Sally about two years of hard work to see herself as anything other than a worthless daughter. During our work together, we identified how Sally tried to protect herself from the negativity her mother embodied. She wasn't a lousy daughter. When she counted down the minutes, she was counting down how much longer she had to diligently maintain her self-protective bubble. Sally struggled significantly with creating boundaries. I've outlined the most potent activity we did together below.

What is one area that you feel you need to be perfect in to be accepted, loved, or respected?

_____

_____

_____

_____

Who do you compare yourself to when you think of yourself as not being perfect?

_____

_____

_____

_____

_____

How are you similar to that person? How are you different?

_____

_____

_____

_____

_____

_____

_____

_____

In what ways are you trying to please this person by becoming something that you are not?

_____

_____

_____

_____

_____

_____

_____

Boundaries are essential for addressing our tendencies toward perfection. Use this activity to identify your boundaries. Draw a house as if you had removed the roof and looked down into the house. You may make this drawing as elaborate or barren as you want. Some of my clients say they have no artistic ability and draw a square with a break in the lines for a "door" and a "window," while others will be quite elaborate and design their dream home!

As you continue this activity, leave the space by the front door blank.

Write your boundaries on the outside of the house. What emotions, thoughts, and actions do you want to keep **out** of your life? Be honest, even if you think these boundaries may hurt someone else. Often, we don't set limits out of deference to others' feelings, so we pay the price ourselves.

Now on the inside of the house, write the emotions, thoughts, and actions you want in your life.

Look at your house. Do you see a representation of your life? If you do, then good! That's what we need. If not, edit it until you do.

Now for the most pivotal part of this assignment. Outside of the front door, list the people you do not want to let in right now (or ever). On the inside of the door, list who you welcome into your circle. If you have people, you consider conditional— meaning that they can sometimes come in and sometimes not— write them directly on the door.

Hang this picture up where you can see it daily. Over time, you might add or remove items. Our boundaries can change as our relationships shift with ourselves and others.

Now just because you have outlined your boundaries doesn't mean that everyone around you will suddenly respect them. You will need to find and use your voice repeatedly to ensure that others respect your wishes. Sometimes this will be easier than others, but with time and practice you will become more adept. Hold fast to your voice. If that doesn't work, you can always walk away! Driving yourself crazy, trying to control people and situations, fuels negativity and destroys progress.

Perfectionism will drive you crazy. Trying the same things repeatedly to become someone else only ever produces negative results. For those who genuinely love you, it's misery watching you constantly berate and belittle the fantastic person you are.

Crazy eventually turns cruel and then crazy again. We figure we can achieve perfection if we can be just a little more "disciplined." Except discipline isn't favorable in this case. It's what drives us to loathe ourselves a little bit more each minute. It's a herd of gremlins telling us that we're not good enough.

To combat those tough moments, return to mindfulness and living in the present moment. If depression is living in the past, and anxiety is trying to control the future, where are you? It takes work to live in the present moment and savor the right now. The past tempts our minds to worry over the what-ifs. The future challenges us to control it—we just have to look the right way, have the ideal job, or raise the best kids. (Easily done, right?)

Take a moment and list everything in this moment that you are grateful for or think you are doing well.

_____

_____

_____

_____

_____

_____

_____

_____

_____

_____

_____

_____

Each day spend time focusing on the functional areas in your life instead of the ones you feel are a mess. When you recognize strategies that create positivity, you can apply those strategies to the places you want to improve. The goal is to become the best you, not impersonate the person next to you.

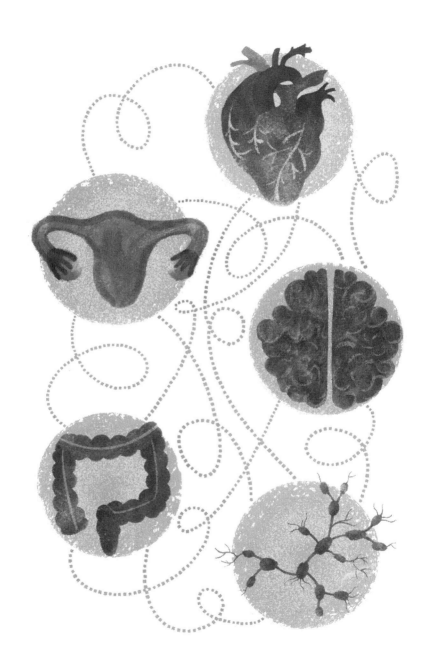

5 Systems and 5 Thoughts

*The Doctor of the future will give no
medication, but will interest his patients in the
care of the human frame, diet and in the
cause and prevention of disease.*

—Thomas A. Edison

Section 1: The Gut (Gastrointestinal tract)

Trust your gut

1. Let go!
2. Gettin' buggy wit' it!
3. Soothing the beast.

The gastrointestinal tract, also known as the gut or intestines, is much like life. Each person's abdomen houses approximately 20 feet of intestines between the small and large intestines combined. Can you believe that any organ in your body is that long? To fit in the small space of our stomachs, the intestinal tract must twist, turn and lie upon itself, much like our own lives.

How many times have you thought that your life would go one way only to have it take an abrupt twist? Some people find this exciting, but for most of my clients, it causes great stress. Many people I work with hold their pasts and stresses in their gut. Then they become constipated, rundown, lethargic, and some eventually develop autoimmune conditions.

When I was about 13-years-old, I started experiencing all sorts of gastrointestinal issues. I was *drinking* an anti-diarrhea medication and alternating between constipation and diarrhea! My body was never happy, no matter what foods I ate or avoided. In response, I starved myself all day to avoid having to run to the bathroom during school.

I tried to make some connections by journaling my foods. I couldn't find any consistency so I had no idea what caused the upset. I trusted those around me to buy healthy foods. They tried their best, but I now realize they had no idea how our food supply might damage my intestinal tract.

My emotional angst added to the confusion, making it impossible to diagnose what caused my gut disturbances. I can now identify what I didn't consider then—STRESS! I allowed my emotions to consume me from the inside. As I pushed the emotions deep down into my gut and tried to ignore them, they found a way to make their presence known.

What could stress out a 13-year-old? Two words: *perfection* and *abandonment*. I experienced abandonment at an early age, and it rooted deep within me. I figured if I could be perfect, then it would never happen again. I tried to be perfect for my teachers by wracking my brain and getting the best grades in the class. Someone else always outperformed me. I tried to be perfect for my grandparents at home, changing my personality to please them. Nothing I did ever felt good enough. I tried to be perfect for my peers, going out for any sport that would take me. I wanted to fit in with any crowd so that I wasn't a loner. I even considered trying out for cheerleading to gain entrance into that crowd. Fortunately, I didn't go through with it, since I hated wearing skirts!

Instead, I ate everything that made me feel good at the moment. I stuffed my emotions with processed junk food that irritated my gut and triggered a cascade of wiring that led to a gut-brain disconnection instead of connection. I was gassy, bloated, and alternated between constipation and diarrhea. Stress added to the imbalanced gut health, and the continued stuffing of emotions made it worse. It was like being stuck in some funhouse loop covered in slime. I couldn't get up and out, no matter how I tried.

I tried everything to be perfect. The only problem was that I was **not** perfect. **No One** is! Not me, not you, not the person next to you while you read this. We can, however, be our own best. This is what I try to coach my clients into realizing. The act of comparison is simply that: an act! You have the power to ditch the script if you want to!

The question then becomes, do *you* want to?

At one point or another, we all have to answer this question. We can continue on the path determined by the narratives we received as children and young adults, dragging our heavy luggage as we go. Or, we can choose a different direction and leave the bags at a crossroads. This is the power of choice.

I could have let my past destroy me. When I was 4-years-old, my father left my ailing mother and me to fend for ourselves. My mother received a lupus (SLE) diagnosis at 18, and at 28, she died from complications. By the time I turned five years old, my shaky world had made insecurity my new middle name. I was fortunate to have family take me in. Some children in my situation ended up moving back and forth from foster families to group homes. If this was you, I am sorry! No child should have had to live that way, and you deserved much more out of life. You can make it so. Sometimes we have to become our own parents in order to get where we want to be. It teaches, shapes, and molds us into great human beings as long as we let it.

This reminds me of a story I once heard. A farmer had an old donkey that had a hard time seeing. One day, it fell into a deep hole. The farmer and his neighbors tried to get the donkey out, but all their efforts failed. The donkey cried over his hopeless situation; sure, he'd die there. The farmer continued to care for the donkey, dropping food in so it would not starve. After a few days, the farmer had a brilliant idea! He grabbed his shovel and began to dump dirt into the hole. The donkey brayed loudly, thinking the farmer intended to bury him alive. The donkey refused to allow this, and with each shovelful, it stepped onto the added soil. Eventually, it could jump out of the hole on its own.

The donkey could have given up and allowed the farmer to bury it. Instead, it made a choice, stepped up on each shovelful of dirt, and got out.

You could choose to allow life to bury you alive. You could give in to the negativity and the pain that you have experienced, but you do not have to. You have a choice—we all do. We can let the stress, hurt, anger, and fear bury us alive one shovel at a time, or we can step up each time life shovels its dirt on us. The choice is always ours!

Some will be able to let the past go. For others, that past is all that is known, and some can only let go a tiny piece at a time. I wish I could ask a quick question to induce that AH-HA! moment that allows you to lay those burdens down. Unfortunately, that question doesn't exist.

Letting go is a personal path, one we can each find through meditation or guided imagery. One note of caution here for anyone who has been diagnosed with depression or suspects they may be depressed: meditation can make depression worse. Please do not attempt meditation without the supervision of your healthcare practitioner.

I find most beginners prefer guided imagery. It provides a foundation for those who are just beginning to let go. You can take advantage of many online videos and recordings. These free resources can help alleviate concerns about finances. One less thing!

As you choose to set a burden down, you may notice the negative voices or gremlins getting louder. They will present the illusion that your healthiest option is to stay where you are. The more discouraged you feel, the more likely you will buy into that false message. This is actually a hard-wired self preservation mechanism that our caveman ancestors passed down to us. Staying where you were at was safe. Staying in the cave kept you alive. It can be overcome, but the first step is to recognize when you are thinking this way and choosing to stay stuck in your current situation.

When this occurs, take a moment and notice. Only notice; don't respond. Hold back. Notice the words the gremlin spews at you. Notice the tone. We can't defeat what we can't see, so construct a mental image of your gremlin. Where is it? What is it doing?

The gremlin knows it will win so long as you can't see it, so it lives in the darkest recesses of your mind. It hides in the shadows of your self-esteem and worth, hoping to remain unseen because you can't win if you don't know what you are up against.

It doesn't mean that you *can't* win. It means you have to outsmart the gremlin.

That means you have to outsmart yourself. When you pause and notice what you say to yourself, you can then change your harmful thoughts and misguided beliefs. You can bend your thoughts to believe anything if you tell yourself something often enough.

So, set a burden down! Which one will you pick? Which one are you most tired of carrying with you?

_____

_____

_____

_____

_____

_____

When you set it down, your gremlin will try to get you to pick it up again. Here is where your power of noticing will come into play. When you recognize the gremlin's influence, stop for a moment and imagine yourself running back to where you dropped your burden. I like to picture my burden dumped in one of those big metal trash cans I see in parks. I like these because they have a covering to prevent animals from getting into them. Once something is inside the trash can, it's far more difficult to retrieve. Picture what works for you, but make it either difficult to get into or so gross that you would never willingly dig in there to get that burden back.

Peer in and look at your burden. What does it look like? What does it smell like? Do you want to carry it around again?

Now, imagine yourself walking away from that trash can. Imagine the trash can melting into the ground behind you, taking the burden with it.

When you catch yourself wanting to pick that burden back up, no matter how often it happens, picture yourself back at that disgusting trash can. Leave the heavy burden there and look around. Try to identify the trigger that prompted you to retrieve it.

If you can avoid the triggers, great! If you can't, then the ability to identify them will give you power over the situation. You can choose to pick the burden up again or leave it where it is. Choices are powerful!

* * *

I remember looking at my family like they were completely nuts when they told me it was better to give than to receive. I was a kid. I wanted to receive all the time! Birthday, Christmas, Hanukkah, Easter, Valentine's, etc. were all holidays that I got to receive! And I was never opposed to gifts between the holidays, either! I found, though, that I did enjoy giving. I loved seeing the expression on someone's face when they received my gift. Their positivity often influenced me, and I would walk away feeling warm inside, knowing I brightened someone's day. I had turned my attention outside of myself, and you know what? The less I focused on my problems, the less my stomach hurt. Through giving, I received in unexpected ways. I made it a priority to give a little something as frequently as I could.

What will be your first gift, and to whom?

_____

_____

_____

Remember to give from a place of positive intention. Give for the sake of giving. It will make the gift (and what you receive) so much sweeter!

Ironically, many of my clients have a challenging time receiving. Often, they equate receiving with weakness, and they see weakness as an imperfection. Oh, that facade of perfection follows us everywhere! And, for many, when they feel the emotions of shame, disappointment (in self), and defeat, those emotions are shoved deep into the gut where they can cause all kinds of trouble. Constipation, diarrhea, stomach aches, etc. are all a possible symptom of buried emotions. Instead of receiving the love and care we need during our struggles, we tend to become like an island and push people away. When was the last time you were able to receive openly without feeling uncomfortable?

Addressing gut health also requires understanding the microbiome. Over the past few years, researchers have found a connection between the levels of gut bacteria and emotional/mental health conditions such as anxiety, schizophrenia, depression, bipolar disorder, etc. Amazing! Could we lessen the mental health crisis by addressing the whole person and looking at how a person's gut processes and absorbs nutrients?

Without going too much into the gut's biochemistry (I did the suffering, so you don't have to. You can thank me later!), every person's gut contains three general categories of bacteria: beneficial (good), opportunistic (bad), and commensal (neutral).

We'll get to the commensal bacteria later. For now, just remember it lives in our guts. The beneficial and harmful bacteria, however, play a large role in our well-being.

Simply put, we want higher levels of good bacteria than bad but all must stay within limits or even too much good can turn bad. The good bacteria help our bodies fight illnesses, food poisoning, and emotional disturbances. It can also help us sleep better. When the harmful bacteria outnumber the good, we are more prone to stomach bugs and emotional disturbances. Our sleep sucks! Sometimes we grow severely ill, as in the cases of autoimmune conditions.

The foods we eat affect our bacteria levels. A diet high in refined carbohydrates creates ideal conditions for the harmful bacteria to flourish, as it feeds on the sugar content. This leads to imbalances in some of the critical feel-good neurotransmitters, such as serotonin. Serotonin is the precursor to melatonin, which among many other things, helps us fall and stay asleep. Sounds pretty important, right? It is!

Want to check your levels? I highly recommend the GI-Map to assess them. It will also look for yeast and parasites while checking for autoimmune markers. (To obtain a GI-Map test kit, please reach out to me or check you with your healthcare provider.)

Once you have your test results, return to this section for further exploration.

What recommendations did your doctor and nutritionist give to rebalance your microbes? Take a moment to write them here:

_____

_____

_____

_____

_____

_____

To which part of the recommendations might you have a hard time adhering?

_____

_____

_____

_____

_____

_____

_____

What part or parts of the recommendations seems doable?

_____

_____

_____

_____

_____

_____

_____

What emotions do you have regarding making the suggested changes?

_____

_____

_____

_____

_____

_____

Emotions play a significant impact on a healthy and properly functioning GI system. To illustrate, allow me to share a personal story. As I write this, I am sitting on an airplane on my way to Utah to meet a sister I never knew I had. Talk about nerve-racking! I have spent all 39 years of my life as an only child, and in an instant, I discovered I'm a younger sister, an aunt, and a great aunt. It is a crazy feeling. I have so many emotions competing for attention, but mostly I am scared to death! Unfortunately, everything that causes me distress also shuts down my digestive system. I woke up with a swollen abdomen, a bit of nausea, no appetite, and we will stop there.

Many others also internalize stress and feel the same signs of sluggish digestion. Here we see the connection between our guts and our emotional minds. A strong relationship between our gut health and our emotional health exists and, yet, the medical community mostly ignores the connection. When I am working with someone who has GI issues such as Crohn's disease, IBS/IBD, arthritis, lupus, celiac, fibromyalgia, or chronic fatigue, to name a few, we also take the time to address underlying stuffed emotions.

So how do we deal with those times when our emotions get the best of us?

If you're like me, you will want to look within and develop a plan to handle the situation. Or perhaps you prefer to recruit a friend, a family member, or an online community to empathize and sympathize with your problem. Which method is better? Only you can make that decision. What research does show, though, is that people with at least one confidant have fewer health issues. Wow! Talk about a powerful antidote to what ails us!

Sadly, less than half of all Americans have someone with whom they feel comfortable confiding. With roughly 327 million people in the US, that is a large number of people who think they have to do things alone. I was one of them, and I struggled through the self-shaming that kept me from identifying with other people and creating a bond.

I have been blessed in the last few years to have found someone who I can call my friend. Aubrey helped me realize I gained nothing by swimming between the islands of self-pity and self-loathing. There are times when I still feel like an island, and at these times, I pick up the phone and send out a signal that I need some help.

Even our gastrointestinal systems have systems of "friendship" within them, which brings us to the commensal bacteria. They live in a symbiotic relationship with our guts. Our nutrient intake nourishes them, and they help convert foods into useful byproducts used by other body systems. Think of commensal bacteria as a valued friend. We support it with nutrients, and it sustains us by keeping other systems healthy.

Without supportive connections during times of distress, we are more likely to feel those stresses on a physical level. The gut is the most commonly affected system. If left unattended, the effects of stress spread to other areas, such as the cardiovascular system, and results in symptoms such as high cholesterol, high blood pressure, heart attack, and stroke. It all started at stress—physical, mental, emotional, or some twisted combination of all three.

We cannot address the things we do not think about or see. You know what is coming next, don't you?

What are some of the stresses you carry in your gut?

_____

_____

_____

_____

_____

_____

Which are the top two most concerning stresses?

_____

_____

_____

_____

_____

_____

What are you willing to do about it?

_____

_____

_____

_____

_____

_____

We can never entirely remove stress from our bodies. Actually, we wouldn't want to because stress forces the body to respond and ensure its systems function correctly. When we have chronic, uncontrolled stress, our bodies struggle to respond appropriately, and they begin to shut down and experience disease.

Think about the word disease. If we break it into its two syllables, we have dis-ease, meaning the opposite of ease. We need more ease in our lives and less dis-ease (stress).

You have probably been advised at some point to reduce your stress levels. Let me offer that advice again. You need to reduce your stress levels.

What was your first emotional reaction to hearing that? if you are anything like my clients, you just turned the stress dial up, not down. Most stress out! How in the world am I going to reduce my stress when I barely have time to think let alone act?

Take a step back for a moment and breathe. How about we change the word *reduce* to *transform*? If I say we need to work on *transforming* your stress levels, does that sound less intimidating? Less like climbing an icy mountain in bedroom slippers?

We all have stress. We cannot avoid it, and in many cases—like the single mother who works two jobs to make ends meet—she cannot reduce her stress. However, we can all transform our stress. Look at these examples, then come up with ones that fit your life.

Instead of eating that cheesecake in the fridge, go for a nice brisk walk—with or without music.

Transform your irritability by painting or journaling about what is bothering you.

Participate in a new hobby—one that will take your mind away from the situation.

Talk to yourself—look in the mirror and ask yourself what is bothering you about your situation and what you are willing to do about it.

What steps can I take to transform my stress so that my gut can rest?

_____

_____

_____

_____

_____

_____

What am I willing to do at this moment?

_____

_____

_____

_____

_____

_____

It is also essential to address what we are not able to do at this moment. We simply cannot be all things—even to ourselves—at all times. This part of the process helps us identify what is and is not feasible.

What are some of the limitations that you have in transforming your stress?

_____

_____

_____

_____

_____

_____

Are they really limitations, or are they excuses?

_____

_____

For any that are excuses, take a moment to rewrite them into positive action steps instead.

Example: I can't because I have no time. (Excuse)

Example: I realize my time is limited, I'm willing to sacrifice

_____ in my schedule in order to make

_____ a priority. (Positive Action Step)

_____

_____

_____

_____

_____

_____

_____

_____

_____

_____

_____

_____

_____

Section 2: Cardiovascular System—Loving Yourself Beyond the Pain (& Inflammation) and Getting to The Heart of the Matter

1. Blood Pressure

2. Cholesterol

3. Inflammation

4. Love & Grudges

In this section, I ask you to monitor your blood pressure. When you check your blood pressure, take care to do so under close to the same circumstances each time as possible. Allow me to explain why.

A typical doctor's appointment begins with the nurse taking readings. You walk back to the examination room, hop onto the infamous paper-lined table, and expose your upper arm for the blood pressure cuff. Efficient nurses use the time to ask questions and speed up your appointment process.

Sounds like a typical medical appointment, so what is wrong with this picture?

First of all, movement triggers a short spike in blood pressure. As we walk to the examination room, our bodies pump oxygen and nutrients to our muscles, so we do not crash to the floor mid-stride. Then we climb up on the table—which requires more energy. Conversation can also raise blood pressure. That's three strikes in two minutes, resulting in inaccurate readings.

Not everyone with a hypertension diagnosis received an incorrect diagnosis. If this were the case, our medical professionals would adjust their practices. However, to effectively identify and interpret blood pressure changes, you need to know what they know and establish a consistent baseline.

Since all their patients make the same walk every visit, nurses can account for that activity. But if you compare your nurse's reading in the office to your reading taken before you get out of bed, your points of comparison lack accuracy. The difference in the two readings would indicate only a change in activity level, not a change in cardiovascular health.

Now that you understand the vital concept of *monitoring* your blood pressure let's dig deeper into *why* I want you to keep track of it.

Your cardiovascular system functions like a loop. The blood fills up with oxygen at the lungs, then travels through the arteries delivering oxygen and nutrients to your many organs. It makes the return trip to the lungs through the veins. Your heart powers the entire operation, keeping the blood moving.

Blood pressure readings indicate how hard your heart has to work to accomplish this. That makes blood pressure an excellent measure of cardiovascular health. If anything gets in the way of the flow of blood, we can experience high blood pressure (hypertension). Blockages and cholesterol are the most common obstacles.

Approximately 75 million Americans are diagnosed with hypertension yearly, and many more go undiagnosed. Hypertensive patients typically manage the condition with pharmaceuticals. Unfortunately, those medications do not address the underlying causes, and the individual remains at risk for developing further complications such as cardiovascular disease, heart attacks, and strokes.

One afternoon, I interviewed about 50 people at a local park, asking them what they thought a regular blood pressure reading was. Most of them quickly told me 120/80. While this is what we have been told is acceptable, it's the highest point before someone is classified pre-hypertensive.

When I weighed 350+ pounds (at just under 5'5"), I had a host of things wrong with me—high cholesterol, poor waist-hip ratio, PCOS, anovulation, hirsutism, and most likely several nutrient deficiencies. I wasn't in a place of good health. I got winded and broke a sweat going up a single flight of stairs. My knees ached from the pressure of hoisting my immense body up the stairs.

At that time, my blood pressure typically read 120-125/80. Now that I've reached a healthy weight, my average blood pressure hovers around 110/68. We must pay attention to our bodies in addition to considering widely accepted medical norms. According to my "normal" reading, my blood pressure was not a problem, but my body knew better. At 120/80, my heart worked harder than others' hearts, and I could feel it.

I urge every woman reading this book to be honest with herself. Do you have difficulty getting up a few stairs? Do you feel other indicators of heart strain? If so, your heart is working overtime, and you need to stake steps to get and keep it healthy. We cannot address that which we refuse to see!

So, let us take a moment and get your baseline. If you do not have a blood pressure monitor at home, you may need to seek the assistance of someone who does or, at the very least, go to your local pharmacy and use the machines that they have tucked away in a corner. Here is what you need to do:

1. Double-check with your nurse, doctor, pharmacist to make sure you have the correct size cuff. Using the wrong size will give you an inaccurate reading.

2. Get positioned in a comfortable spot and sit *quietly* for 5 minutes. No talking or moving, and take some deep breaths to calm your nervous system.

3. Take blood pressure.

4. If you experience dizziness upon standing, also take your blood pressure right after sitting up from a prone (laying down) position. If you do not have a problem with dizziness upon standing, please skip to number 7.

5. Lay quietly for 10 minutes (Minimum of 5 minutes between readings + 5 minutes for quiet time) with the cuff in place but not inflated.

6. Sit up and take blood pressure. **Please do not stand up during this time. Sitting is adequate and significantly safer.

7. Repeat the process for the next two days at roughly the same time each day.

8. Take the average of your blood pressure readings.

For those of you who are doing the prone-position blood pressure measurement because of dizziness, this dizziness can be due to a condition called orthostatic hypotension. It is important to assess your adrenal gland function.

Blood pressure reading:

Day 1:

Sitting _____ Prone _____

Day 2:

Sitting _____ Prone _____

Day 3:

Sitting _____ Prone _____

Average:

Sitting _____ Prone _____

Hypertension and hyperlipidemia often hang out together. Hyperlipidemia— high cholesterol—is like a bear in the woods. We should respect it and heed its warnings, but we know better than to try to chase it away from its home. Yet we often look into its home—the body—and try to eradicate it.

Cholesterol is necessary for the synthesis of vitamin D and the production of hormones. It is meant to be there. Cholesterol can also function like that overly sensitive smoke detector in your kitchen that goes off anytime you boil water!

Elevated cholesterol levels doesn't mean we have a deficiency of a statin drug. More likely, we have an abundance of inflammation. If we force our cholesterol levels down through medications, we allow the inflammation to attack the vital organs that keep us functioning day-to-day. Then what's the best way to balance your cholesterol levels and get them back into the optimally healthy range?

Address the inflammation. Our bodies have a natural inflammation system. In small amounts, inflammation is a good thing. It helps us when we injure ourselves or when we are sick. That inflammation alerts us to a problem and inspires us to take action. However, low-grade, chronic inflammation that arises from constant stress, unaddressed emotions, an improper diet full of low-quality fats and high in sugar, lack of sleep, and lack of exercise leads to increased cholesterol production.

We have all been there. We have all put ourselves last in line when it comes to care, but you can turn that around. First, work with your health care practitioner to identify sources of inflammation. Reduction and removal are essential here. Once you have successfully identified the inflammation sources, you can address them through nutrition, exercise, supplementation, and play! Take a few moments and survey your current lifestyle. What are some of the inflammation sources that you can identify on your own? Do you smoke? Do you drink? Do you live a relatively sedentary life where you spend more time sitting than anything else? Are you plagued by negative thought patterns about yourself, your life, or the world around you?

My Sources of Inflammation:

Physical: _____

_____

_____

_____

_____

_____

Mental: _____

_____

_____

_____

_____

_____

Social: _____

_____

_____

_____

_____

_____

Emotional: _____

_____

_____

_____

_____

If you get overwhelmed by the number of inflammation sources, remember you don't have to tackle all at once. That might backfire by increasing your stress and causing more inflammation! Pick one source in each group and start there. Expand as you feel able.

Often in my practice, I find that my clients have been holding on to anger and are, at times, reluctant to identify and work through it. For some, it's a matter of not knowing how the anger will be expressed. They fear hurting themselves or others with all of the stuffed anger. The problem isn't the anger itself. It's that we don't know what to do with anger. It is incredibly scary for us women as we are taught not to be angry. Instead, we are taught to always be sweet and kind. Screw that! We have anger, too! We are allowed to be upset with those who have hurt us or situations that didn't go as we intended. We are entitled to scream, punch our fists into a pillow (but never each other!), cry, or go inward to process this very intense and often overwhelming feeling. When we don't allow ourselves to "befriend" the emotion of anger, we often end up holding a grudge. These grudges also create an emotional imbalance that leads to the development of inflammation.

Successful people don't hold grudges, yet it's difficult for many people to let grievances go. We want to defend them by making the case that they help us. We use grudges to protect ourselves or as motivationalk fuel. Society has conditioned us to behave and think this way.

Let's take a moment to walk through this activity. Complete it first by recalling a grudge you held but have since resolved.

The Grudge that Won't Budge Activity

Recall a situation in which you held a grudge against someone (or a group).

Who was the person or group?

_____

When did the situation take place?

_____

What was said or done?

_____

_____

_____

_____

_____

How did it make you feel?

_____

_____

_____

_____

_____

What did you learn about yourself?

_____

_____

_____

_____

_____

_____

_____

_____

_____

What did holding on to the hurt and anger do to you *mentally?*

_____

_____

_____

_____

_____

What did holding on to the hurt and anger do to you *emotionally?*

_____

_____

_____

_____

_____

_____

_____

_____

_____

_____

_____

What did holding on to the anger do to you *physically*?

_____

_____

_____

_____

_____

_____

_____

_____

_____

_____

_____

_____

How did **you** holding on to the anger affect the other person/ people?

_____

_____

_____

_____

_____

Who suffered by you holding on to the anger? (I'll give you a hint, it's not the people you listed at the beginning.)

_____

Now for the hard part. Go back through that activity using a current grudge. I know we've already spoiled the ending, but you can use the perspective you gained through hindsight to analyze the present.

What do you do with this information now that we have dredged it up? Let go! UGH! So easy for me to say, but more difficult to do. Yes, no greater a truth has ever been spoken. However, you have the power in your hands. You are stronger today than the day you picked up this book. You can do anything, and if you continue to hold on to the hurt and anger, your mental, emotional and physical symptoms will only worsen.

Letting go is easier said than done, so here are some suggestions to help you along this process. Keep in mind that letting go doesn't happen overnight. Please be patient with yourself and learn to forgive yourself in those moments that you backslide.

1. Write a letter to the person/people who hurt you. At the end of the message, in the center, write in BIG, **BOLD** letters: **"I FORGIVE YOU, AND I AM LETTING THIS GO. NO MORE ANGER. NO MORE HURT. I LOVE ME TOO MUCH TO HOLD ON TO THIS ANY LONGER."** Mailing it or handing it to the person is an option, but burning it, burying it, tearing it up, dancing on it, or any other destructive activity type would work as well. This activity is about you, so have at it.

2. Release through breath—Sit in a safe, comfortable place and focus on your breathing. Take long, deep inhalations, filling your belly. As you continue to take long breaths, I want you to focus on breathing into your heart. Deep breathing may

be tricky at first, but keep practicing, and you will eventually learn to visualize the breath filling your heart cavity. Your heart comes online and feels emotions much faster than your brain does. Therefore, inhaling into the heart allows it to have the oxygen that it needs to perform correctly, but it also brings in love, calmness, and appreciation into your heart. You may also take this time to imagine a moment or a person in your life that resembles love, peace, and gratitude.

3. Engage in an enjoyable physical activity. Although it isn't your only option, running is a popular choice because it lends itself easily to metaphor. Our grudges come from the past. We can't change what happened, so we look at the present and to the future. Visualize your goal, the end picture you want to obtain, off in the distance. Now start running. Focus your intention on that positive image, and don't look back. While this might feel like "running" from your problems or your past, that is not the intent here. You have been trying to run from your problems by holding an emotion and by not addressing the situation or allowing yourself the space to experience your feelings. Focus not on running from problems or the past. Instead, run toward positivity—running toward release and happiness. By running toward your future, you automatically distance yourself from your history.

4. Indulge your creativity—find something you enjoy doing that allows you to express hurt and anger. Paint, draw, color, or sculpt it out. I loved to paint and sacrificed many canvases in my younger years (and sometimes still today) to broad, aggressive strokes of bold, dark colors. I assign colors to my emotions and see what happens on the canvas. For those

who don't lean toward the visual arts, creativity comes in many flavors. Perhaps you create through music, crafting, or writing.

5. Take a bath. Add some Epsom salts and essential oils (my favorites are lavender and grapefruit together) to the bathwater. Soak. Imagine the water cleansing the hurt and anger from your body. You might also use bath time to work with activity number 2. When you're ready, exit the tub before draining the water. Imagine all of the negativity that washed off of you floating in the bathwater and release the plug. As the water washes your grudge down the drain, you may say a little prayer, a chant, or anything that comes to your mind as you release the negativity and watch it swirl down the drain.

6. Activity of your choice. What is a non-food related activity that brings you solace? What do do when you need a moment of peace? Document it here in case you wish to return to it when you recognize a new grudge to release.

_____

_____

_____

_____

_____

_____

_____

_____

_____

_____

_____

_____

Complete this section after you have completed your chosen activity.

What did you learn about yourself during this process?

_____

_____

_____

_____

_____

_____

_____

_____

_____

_____

_____

Are there any feelings left unaddressed during this time?

_____

_____

_____

_____

_____

_____

If so, how might you best address them?

_____

_____

_____

_____

_____

_____

Remember, behind a grudge lies anger, hurt, or disappointment. Most humans seek to avoid these unpleasant feelings—or at least stuff them so far down that we no longer feel them. No matter how much we try to prevent or suppress anger, hurt, and disappointment, our physical bodies will continue to feel them. Sadly, we can develop a multitude of disease states as a result. That deep pain in our hearts is a warning sign—a plea—to let go.

When we learn to let go—we learn to fly.

Section 3: Endocrine—Balancing Precariously on the Edge

Balance

1. Adrenal Hormones

2. Sex Hormones

3. Thyroid Hormones

I once heard a presenter liken hormones to toddlers. They need constant supervision and are prone to distraction. I now incorporate this simple yet compelling explanation into almost all of my clients' plans to help them understand the root of their imbalances.

Our hormones have such a profound impact on who we are, what we think, what we look like, and how we perceive ourselves. Women tend to understand this, thanks to our cycles. What changes do you see when you compare yourself mid-cycle to a week after it has ended? These changes—anything from irritability and sleeplessness to increased sex drive and bloating—result from our fluctuating hormones.

Many of my clients come to me as a last resort. They know something is wrong, but blood tests come back normal—leaving them confused as to why they feel out of balance but are told they are fine. They are tired of being labeled as crazy when they insist they don't feel well. Each of us has our "normal." We measure hormones in ranges, rarely absolutes. No lab test could prove that we are or aren't normal.

We ladies have carried the crazy label as far back as 1900BC. Accusations against women included irrationality, hallucinations, and emotional outbursts. Society much prefers a well-poised, quiet and timid woman rather than one who expresses her thoughts, opinions, and emotions. Some insane theories have resulted from this belief in hysteria (think wandering wombs and doctors providing orgasmic pelvic massages).

When our hormones get out of balance, we genuinely feel crazy, which can affect our actions. If we understand how to remediate these hormonal imbalances, we can start to feel normal again. However, this doesn't always happen immediately. Many times, we are simply told that what we are feeling is all in our heads. We are left with more questions as we walk out of the practitioner's office. Over and over, we may face this challenge. If this is you, please don't feel like you are alone. I spent many hours in various doctor's offices trying to get a diagnosis for my PCOS. Something that I would later come to know as common eluded doctors in their diagnosis. Instead, they blamed my weight. It was a message that I heard many times. Do not give up! Since I have been in the proverbial shoes of the "crazy hypochondriac," I can all also empathize with how you are feeling. What I can say is that this too shall pass! Managing the emotions requires hormone rebalance. So, when you feel out of control, your hormones may be the real culprit.

Stress can make us feel even crazier when we can't seem to handle even the simplest of tasks. In the previous section, we addressed how stress can damage the heart by creating a low-grade, chronic inflammation. Here, we will talk about stress's impact on hormones, primarily through cortisol, produced by the adrenal gland.

Over the last decade or so, stress reduction has become a huge conversation piece. It's on the news. It's in the magazines. Doctors are talking about it. But what is the big deal? Everyone has stress in their lives, right? Absolutely! It's what you do with it that counts. We can never live a stress-free experience. The reality is that our bodies need to have some stress to force it to grow, regenerate, and adapt to our environments. Not having stress can be equally as dangerous as having too much. In all things, we balance.

So instead of wishing that all stress would just disappear and we could sit on the beach every day sipping fruity cocktails with pretty little paper umbrellas, we seek to transform the stressors from negative to positive. Let's take a look at the following scenario:

Mary was up all night arguing with her husband over who would stay home to care for their sick son, Micah. Mary always lost that battle, so she arrived to work 45 minutes late. She missed an important meeting, and her boss spent an hour yelling at her.

Since the week she discovered his affair, Mary has wanted to leave her husband, but her bank account won't let her go anywhere anytime soon. No matter how many strides she makes at work, it won't provide enough to support herself and her son—especially if the professional sacrifices always fall on her shoulders. After today, she's lucky she even has a job.

But she has no time for reflection. She has to take their son to his two-hour baseball practice, then come home and make dinner while helping him with his homework. After dinner, Mary cleans the kitchen and begins preparing for the next day, ensuring their son practices good hygiene and gets to bed on time.

By the time Mary has a little time to herself, it's after 9 pm, and she still has a full to-do list. She wishes a typical day looked different, but tomorrow will resemble this one. There is never enough time to get everything done. Her shoulders hurt from the constant tension.

Over the last few months, Mary has noticed an increase in her heart palpitations. She also has trouble sleeping. Mary drinks a bit more than she used to and uses sleep aids to quiet her mind so she can fall asleep. Mary knows she needs to figure out a better way.

Can you relate to this story at all? Stress adds up, and, as you can see, Mary's stress affects her physical well-being.

What does your stress story look like? Write it out here. (You may choose to write about one specific stress, a stressful day, or however the stress appears in your life.)

_____

_____

_____

_____

_____

_____

_____

_____

_____

_____

What was the experience like for you while writing out your stress story?

_____

_____

What physical symptoms have you noticed that may be a result of your stress levels?

_____

_____

_____

_____

_____

_____

_____

How many hours do you sleep each night?

_____

Do you tend to eat more or less when you are stressed, worried, or anxious?

_____

What foods do you crave when you are tense?

_____

_____

_____

_____

_____

_____

_____

_____

The Hypothalamus-Pituitary-Adrenal (HPA) axis produces the primary stress hormone cortisol, which helped our prehistoric ancestors avoid being eaten by a bear or a mountain lion. As a response to stress, the adrenal gland should produce a surge of cortisol for a short period and, with rest, return to normal thereafter. However, the calm after the storm does not come as readily as it once did. In our modern lives, we spend more time running to keep up with deadlines and activities. Our ancestors didn't do this. They ran from the bear or saber-tooth tiger and then had a long period of rest. No, I'm not referring to the fact that they got eaten! I'm referring to the time that they spent hiding in their caves chillin' and waiting until they felt it was safe to go back out again. Our current lifestyle, where we run from stressor to stressor without pausing to process what we are feeling or to rest, takes a toll on the HPA axis and our overall health.

Why do we try to fill every minute of every day? Often, it's a distraction attempt. We have something in our lives that we don't want to face, and keeping ourselves busy allows us to avoid it, just like our ancestors avoided those bears.

From what are you running? From what are you trying to escape?

_____

_____

_____

_____

_____

_____

_____

_____

_____

_____

_____

The truth of the matter is that we can't outrun our lives. We also can't change the past. Sometimes bad things happen to help us to appreciate the good in our lives.

I have been raped. For years after, I feared dating. I was afraid of putting myself out there again. I didn't want to go anywhere alone. Heck, I didn't want to go anywhere, period!

Over time, I learned to hide. I stayed in my house more and more. I was skeptical of everyone I met. I blamed myself for what had happened. I had to have *done* something to cause this.

I also hid by keeping busy. I started running. I lifted weights at the gym and battled to the front of the boxing class. I buried myself in work. I stressed myself out by focusing on all of the things that I wasn't doing well. Even my art had to be perfect, or I threw the canvas out. Nothing was ever good enough. Nothing was ever done enough. Nothing was ever perfect enough. Nothing was ever clean enough.

I was never enough.

This concept of not being enough plagues so many of us, and it is, indeed, a huge stressor in our lives.

I know now that I was enough then, and I am enough now, but it has taken me awhile to get to the point that I feel safe sharing this.

You are enough
Just as you are
Right now
No questions and no explanations needed.

Complete these sentences:

I like myself because: _____

_____

_____

_____

_____

_____

_____

I love myself because: _____

_____

_____

_____

_____

_____

_____

_____

I get frustrated with myself when I: _____

_____

_____

_____

_____

_____

_____

_____

I find enjoyment in: _____

_____

_____

_____

_____

_____

_____

_____

A great day would consist of: _____

_____

_____

_____

_____

_____

_____

Today I release myself from: _____

_____

_____

_____

_____

_____

_____

_____

I am *not* responsible for: _____

_____

_____

_____

_____

_____

I *am* responsible for: _____

_____

_____

_____

_____

_____

_____

I will allow myself to think: _____

_____

_____

_____

_____

_____

_____

I will allow myself to feel: _____

_____

_____

_____

_____

_____

The scariest part of letting go is: _____

_____

_____

_____

_____

_____

_____

What I am most looking forward to in this process is: _____

_____

_____

_____

_____

_____

_____

I anticipate these challenges during this process: _____

_____

_____

_____

_____

_____

_____

For each of your challenges, list them here again with a solution next to them.

_____

_____

_____

_____

_____

_____

_____

_____

_____

_____

_____

_____

_____

_____

Sadly, many women share a common experience of trauma. The trauma looks different for each of us, but the result is the same. Our traumas forced us into the overstimulated HPA axis clubhouse. None of us ever wanted to join this club, but if you look around, you will see an extraordinary sisterhood of fighters.

We live in a heightened state of fear of life, partnership, and vulnerability. Our past experiences teach us to distrust and remain on guard. Our fear dictates our lives in a way that nothing else can. It protects us, after all—it keeps us safe on the sidelines, spectators of our own lives.

Even when we feel life is moving along quite nicely, our bodies still keep us alert and on edge.

I have worked with many clients who have insisted they don't feel stressed. Yet, their hormone test results come back with imbalanced cortisol (stress hormone) levels, suggesting that something lies deep below the surface.

Approaching someone about their trauma is never easy. We fiercely guard these sensitive areas, sometimes even blocking out those memories entirely. It's painful. It's ugly. It's unwanted. It's dirty. I've heard it all.

Yes, it is painful, but it's not ugly. Storms cause destruction, but after they clear, we clean up and rebuild under beautiful blue skies. Our storms can either build us or break us.

In the next exercise, I will ask you to write about your traumatic experiences. You will likely find this uncomfortable. That is ok. I have not yet asked you to do anything easy yet so why start now?! By working through this book and getting to this point, you've proven you're committed to change and willing to face discomfort. However, I do want to stress that if you feel that looking at your trauma is too much to face or if it causes you to go to a dark place, skip this section. Please reach out to a local therapist who specializes in PTSD and trauma so that you have someone guiding you.

For those who choose to continue, know that the experiences may rush full blast like a fire hose, or they may trickle like a leaky faucet. Either is fine, but whatever you do, let them flow.

Which of your past experiences is affecting you today?

_____

_____

_____

_____

_____

_____

_____

_____

What would it take for you to lay this experience down or change your perspective of it?

_____

_____

_____

_____

_____

_____

_____

Who do you need to forgive during this time?

_____

_____

_____

_____

For what do they need forgiveness?

_____

_____

_____

_____

_____

_____

How can you forgive yourself for holding on to this trauma?

_____

_____

_____

_____

_____

_____

_____

_____

_____

_____

_____

_____

_____

_____

The concept of forgiving ourselves for our past trauma can seem weird. We were the victim in the situation, after all. Someone took something from us or did something to us without our consent. Their actions cost us in that moment, but if we allow that person to continue taking from us, they impede our ability to live a full, happy and healthy life.

Here is where self-forgiveness comes into play. We have to forgive ourselves for the time and energy we've given to our fear, anger, and hurt. When we learn to recognize old thought patterns that no longer serve us, we honor ourselves. We foster self-confidence and love instead of self-doubt and loathing.

* * *

The HPA axis—our adrenals—function in tandem with the sex hormones (estrogen, testosterone, and progesterone). They rely on each other to maintain an internal balance within the body. When the body stays in fight-or-flight mode, cortisol remains activated. The sex hormones, considered nonessential by the body under stressful situations, get left behind until the stress passes. Pharmaceuticals can force the sex hormones to appear balanced. This often happens in cases like Polycystic Ovary Syndrome, where birth control pills force the body to menstruate, yet the underlying cause of the sex hormone imbalance remains unaddressed or is ultimately worsened. Our bodies can go on functioning this way for a while, but not forever. Eventually, the adrenals become exhausted, our ability to respond to stress declines, and the production of our sex hormones takes a further hit.

Let's make an inventory of the things you enjoy but no longer make time for. _____

_____

_____

_____

_____

What gets in the way of you spending time participating in these activities?

_____

_____

_____

_____

Which of those things above can you eliminate or reduce?

_____

_____

_____

_____

What day(s) of the week could make time to indulge in some favorite pastimes?

_____

What, if any, obstacles might impede making time for the activities?

_____

_____

_____

_____

_____

How can you overcome these obstacles?

_____

_____

_____

_____

_____

_____

As we learn to transform our stress from a negative view to a more positive perspective, our HPA axis can relax and allow our hormones to balance. Doing so requires our stress transformation activities and possibly supplements, as well. While supplements can support our progress, they don't do the hard work for us. We must make significant changes, including mindfulness, following a proper diet, loving ourselves, and allowing ourselves space to heal.

Trauma is a detrimental HPA axis disruptor we can easily conceal. In response to trauma, we busy ourselves caring for others. We bury our hurts, push through to the next activity, and force ourselves to continue as if nothing happened. But that incest, rape, abuse, and neglect, doesn't ever go away. It becomes part of the tapestry of our life. We bury it deeply and try to forget it, but we stay in a constant, heightened alert. Loud noises scare us. We regularly check over our shoulders, trusting no one and fearing almost everyone. We find it challenging to accept a touch. We hate our bodies, loathing their feminine softness or distinctly feminine scent. We can even develop conditions such as fibroids, PCOS, endometriosis, and infertility.

Does the idea of trauma contributing to your hormonal imbalance resonate? While this book's scope cannot walk you through your trauma, it is essential to identify and address these issues. Leaving them unchecked impedes our bodies' ability to balance hormones, conceive a child, and maintain overall health.

*　*　*

The almost daily roller coaster of emotions caused by our hormone fluctuations can feel daunting, even downright debilitating. When our hormones are in balance, we feel good, as if we could take on the world and succeed at anything. When they are out of balance, we feel stress more intensely, and we cope less easily. Our hair falls out or grows where we don't want it. Our weight fluctuates.

The sex hormones also affect how we view ourselves as sexual beings. When they are in balance, we can be on our A-game in the bedroom. When they are out of balance, we feel insecure about our bodies and are less likely to seek an intimate moment.

When we reach out to our doctors, they often tell us it's merely in our heads. They advise us to lose a few pounds, and then everything will fall into place. But what happens when it doesn't? What happens when you still feel like crap even after you lost some weight?

You aren't crazy. The answer isn't always a superficial one. What you feel is your experience, and you are entitled to feel it—all of it.

When the HPA axis is disrupted or inflamed, the adrenal glands struggle to support the balanced production of estrogen, testosterone, and progesterone. So often is the case in menopausal and postmenopausal women, whose ovaries produce less estrogen. When I see these women in my practice, often their depleted adrenals can't step in to help out.

You can find all sorts of products designed to bolster the natural production of female sex hormones—over-the-counter, professional supplements, pharmaceuticals. You will know your body is in balance if it remains normalized after you cease taking these products. If your acne returns, your sex drive declines, your hair falls out again, etc., then the products, not your body, were doing the work.

Remember to address the underlying causes and not expect a product to solve the symptoms. You may have heard our health care system in the United States referred to as the sick care system. It helps when the situation warrants a medication, but until then, it's a watch-and-wait scenario. What if we didn't wait to act until we "required" a medication? Knowing your levels and listening to your body can help you prevent getting to this point. Those tired feelings are only normal if you have been working hard.

Trauma affects the adrenals, and the adrenals affect the sex hormones. Because of this relationship, one of the most common causes of infertility that I see in my practice is trauma—sexual, mental, and physical. Our bodies—sometimes subconsciously—have an uncanny way of inhibiting the life cycle when it senses all is not right. The adrenals also support the production of other sex hormones, especially in postmenopausal women. However, for those who are not there yet, the ovaries are still our primary hormone producers. To keep things understandable here, what you need to know is that DHEA is considered the master hormone produced by the adrenals, the gonads, and the brain. When trauma is present, and the brain and adrenals are busy trying to keep you safe by increasing your cortisol production, we almost always see a reduction in testosterone since DHEA converts to either testosterone or cortisol.

Testosterone governs our sexual desire. When those levels drop— most often through imbalanced cortisol or blood sugar levels—our sexual passion wanes. For some, it's a spinning cycle of not being comfortable in our skin or thinking that there is something fundamentally wrong with who we are or what our bodies look like. While scant scientific studies explore how our thoughts impact our sex hormones specifically, we have evidence that our minds can change our physiology. Think about people who overcome significant illnesses like cancer. Those who have a positive mindset are far more likely to recover than those who don't.

Likewise, those of us who face a sex hormone imbalance need the same positive mindset. When we think our bodies have betrayed us or that we will never achieve balance again, our bodies hear us loud and clear and will answer us by confirming our expectations.

What are some of the negative things you tell yourself about your body?

_____

_____

_____

_____

_____

_____

_____

_____

_____

_____

Select one or two negative thoughts and rewrite them with a positive message. Your internal judge or gremlin is likely to shout quite loudly at you while you do this. Put him/her out of your mind and focus on the truth. Don't worry if this task takes some time and challenges you. Just keep trying!

_____

_____

_____

_____

_____

_____

_____

_____

The thyroid imbalance often occurs in women. Hyperthyroidism, hypothyroidism, and Hashimoto's Autoimmune run rampant in our modern society. Various studies have pointed to the amount of fluoride in our water, toxins in our environment, gluten-sensitivity, or the imbalance of the complex HPA axis overlap with the HPT (Hypothalamus-Pituitary-Thyroid). Thyroid hormone production starts in the brain. Many things can affect thyroid hormone production. However, an exciting concept has slowly emerged from studying the connection between energetic fields and medicine: thyroid imbalance may also come from an inability to speak one's truth.

It's far more socially acceptable for women to avoid rocking the boat. We learn at a young age to keep our mouths shut and suppress any thought or emotion that might upset the peace. As we observe this outer peace that comes as a result of our passivity, a war develops within us and compromises our health. Then, we get understandably frustrated when our own unvoiced needs remain largely unmet even when we're the ones who aren't voicing our concerns.

If you could hold a conversation with one person, past or present, about something that you have held or are holding deep inside, who would you choose, and what would you talk about?

What concerns do you have about the outcome of the conversation?

_____

_____

_____

_____

_____

_____

_____

What emotions come up for you surrounding this conversation?

_____

_____

_____

_____

_____

_____

_____

_____

_____

_____

Sit with your emotions regarding your conversation. What effects do those emotions have on your body? For example, if you are angry, are you shaking? Sweating? Tingling? Struggling to catch your breath? Are you tearful because you feel sad? Do you feel less tense because you are feeling more relieved? What is your body trying to tell you?

_____

_____

_____

_____

_____

_____

_____

_____

_____

_____

_____

_____

What are you most afraid of when you think of letting those emotions happen?

_____

_____

_____

_____

_____

_____

_____

_____

Speak your truth. What is your truth about the situation?

_____

_____

_____

_____

_____

_____

_____

What steps will you take to keep yourself from holding back in a similar situation?

_____

_____

_____

_____

_____

_____

_____

_____

_____

_____

_____

_____

_____

Section 4: Neurological

Connection

1. Emotions

2. Cognition

Diagnosis of emotional and mental disorders continue to rise in our society. While they might have been just as common a couple of centuries ago, only recently have we brought energy and awareness to the mainstream. So, if you have been diagnosed with an imbalance in your mental or emotional health, you are not alone. This section is for you!

It's worth noting at this early stage that our work in this section assumes you have not suffered any physical damage to your brain. Bear in mind that physically unique brains have their own rules, and I encourage you to work with a professional who can provide one-on-one attention your brain needs.

As we've covered previously, our emotions affect our bodily systems and always start at the heart. Because our physical systems work intricately together, what affects one affects another. An emotional effect on one system can cause a chain reaction through our bodies.

With this journal, we have the perfect place to discuss the critical connection between our thought patterns and emotions. Our thought patterns affect our emotions, then our feelings affect our bodily systems, and finally affect our health.

On any given day, take a stroll through the hallways of social media. What do you notice? Your news feed probably looks a great deal like my own. You have friends who post pictures of their "perfect" life, "perfect" marriage, "perfect" family, and "perfect" job. They only post pictures of themselves in proper makeup and styled hair. The same goes for anyone in the images with them.

On the other end of the spectrum, you'll find the group I call the FML (F*ck My Life) crowd. These people post shocking articles and photos about animal mutilation, kidnapped children, the spread of disease, political warfare, religious hatred, and anything else that could lead one to doubt positive energy exists in this bleak world. Misery loves company, and these people want to drag you down to their level of hell.

Two completely different piles of people. Two completely different ways of thinking. Both correct. We live in a time when the facade is strong and the negativity even stronger. Our minds and our bodies pick up on the vibrations around us. The people around us affect our patterns of thinking, and our patterns of thinking affect the way we feel and the way our bodies function.

In other words, our thoughts have the power to create health or to create disease in our bodies.

We rarely find any sort of neutrality on social media, even though that would better reflect our daily lives. So, what benefit does social media have? That depends on how we interact with it. If we are bummed out about our lives, social media will feed that wolf. However, when we can accept our current situations as starting points, social media can help motivate change.

If we think things can get worse, they will. If we can accept where we are instead of beating ourselves up about our choices and our existence, we can make changes to help improve our current situation. What if we started thinking more positively? We might say to ourselves, "This is where I am right now, and I don't want things to get worse. That means my only option is to get better."

I want to clarify what I've asked you to accept. I want you to accept *yourself* in your current situation, not the current situation itself. I don't want you to be okay with a negative situation, but you should love *yourself* in any case. Self-talk is huge. How we talk to ourselves affects our outcomes and realities. If you woke up every day and thought about today's unique possibilities and the opportunities you'll have to love yourself, what might your situation look like? What might change?

At first, you might not see a way to escape your current situation. You may only see a dismal outcome. In these moments, remember the power of your thoughts.

Let's dive in and determine whether your current thoughts contribute to stagnation or transformation.

What do you think of yourself right now?

_____

_____

_____

_____

_____

_____

_____

_____

What words come to mind when I say, "Love yourself?"

_____

_____

_____

_____

_____

_____

_____

_____

_____

_____

_____

What is one thing you wish to change about your current situation?

_____

_____

_____

_____

_____

_____

What do you think it will take for you to make this change?

_____

_____

_____

_____

_____

_____

Is making this change realistic at this time?

_____

Do feelings of doubt creep in? From where are they coming?

_____

_____

_____

_____

_____

_____

_____

_____

_____

_____

_____

How do your doubts affect your mentality and thought patterns about your situation?

_____

_____

_____

_____

_____

_____

_____

_____

_____

To lessen doubt's power over us, we sometimes have to act as though we already have what we want. Typically, we project to the Universe (Higher Power) what we fear. Instead, we should project what we want. When we send out positive, we get positive back. When we send out negative, negative returns to us. Focus on the positive feelings of what your new experience will be like in order to raise your energetic vibration toward the things you want in your life.

Here is a fun activity to try with someone. Find a partner close to your size and strength. Hold your arm directly out to the side of your body, making a ninety-degree angle with your torso. Have your partner gently push down on your arm while you resist. Find the point where your strength matches your partner's.

Once you have established that point, extend your arm again. This time say "yes" as your partner pushes on your arm. You may repeat "yes" as many times as you wish. Did you notice an increase in your strength?

Now, do the opposite and say "no" as your partner pushes on your arm. Chances are your arm went down more quickly.

This simple activity demonstrates the power our words have over us. "Yes" and "no" can trigger different thought patterns and physiological responses. How many times a day do you tell yourself no—that you shouldn't have or do something—or apologized for existing or asking questions?

Many tell themselves no because they feel undeserving. They don't feel worthy of that item, job, promotion, partner, outfit, pair of shoes, etc. They tell themselves they aren't enough or the money would be better spent elsewhere.

If you see yourself in this, know you aren't alone. Women commonly feel this lack of self-worth, and too few women feel worthy of achieving their life's desires. Society conditions us to give to everyone else, to feel unfulfilled, and to keep our mouths shut about it. No more, ladies!

If you have a history of believing you will fail regardless of the circumstances, you've likely rewired your neurotransmitters to ensure you accomplish these negative ideas. Don't worry; I bring good news. Through your thoughts, you have the power to rewire your brain and become who you want.

* * *

The saying goes, "It is better to give than to receive." Who made up that shit anyway? While giving brings us joy, so does receiving. It's just sometimes harder to accept the gifts and compliments than it is to provide them. Giving is emotionally safer for the most part. Receiving makes us feel vulnerable. For example, I remember the first time my great grandmother told me, "Jennie, you know that giving is the best way to make a woman happy." I was nine. Seriously? A nine-year-old wants to receive, but I felt instantly guilty for it. My great grandmother had just told me that my femininity made it wrong for me to want to receive. This concept trickled over to tangible presents and also into the way I received love. I felt I should give love easily but not receive it. Feeling this way made it impossible for people to return the love I so desperately gave them, and some even took advantage of the situation and abused that love.

Many women struggle to receive a simple compliment. Think about the last time a coworker, a loved one, a friend, or a random passerby on the street complimented your outfit, your hair, your smile, or whatever else. How did you respond? Did you feel a bit flustered? Embarrassed? Awkward? Did you believe this person was telling the truth, or did you suspect they might be patronizing you to get something in return?

Why is it so hard for us women to receive a compliment? To start answering that question, consider how our society often unconsciously interprets compliments as sexual advances. We can't possibly offer or receive one without a sexual undertone.

My wife calls me beautiful all the time, but I still find it difficult to accept. One day, as we lay in bed together, she asked me to call myself beautiful. It felt downright impossible. She hovered over me, pinning my legs beneath her and holding my arms outstretched. She looked into my eyes and told me to say, "I'm beautiful."

I felt like all oxygen had left my body, and I couldn't breathe or speak. I wanted to cry. I wanted the bed to swallow me whole.

She hadn't cornered me to cause discomfort, even though I felt uncomfortable. A challenging aspect of trusting someone completely—whether friend or lover—is to accept that they can see parts of you that you choose to disregard. I saw myself as ugly, and I had silenced the part of myself that could see otherwise. This type of thinking also affected my sense of self-worth, and I viewed myself as unworthy. My partner recognized this and wanted me to see myself through her eyes. It took her threatening to leave the room to get me to squeak out:

"I . . . AM . . . BEAUTIFUL."

That moment changed something, and I started to see myself a little—just a little—differently. Remember, even the tiniest step forward still counts as progress. We only delay progress when we go backward.

I cried in her arms, wondering how I would ever overcome years of hearing that I was fat, ugly, and worthless. I realized that I possessed great weapons to fight against my inner demons. I had my strengths and also the support of someone who could love me beyond my pain.

The inability to or discomfort around receiving love (in any form) is a learned behavior and can be unlearned.

Achieving significant changes in our thinking is far more problematic when we try to do it alone. Go back to chapter 4 and look at your support system again. Who in your group do you feel comfortable trusting with the dirtiest jobs—helping you address the negative thought tapes that lurk in your mind?

_____

What will his or her role be?

_____

_____

_____

_____

_____

_____

How will this individual hold you accountable for the change that you are trying to make?

_____

_____

_____

_____

_____

Are there any boundaries to which you want this individual to adhere? Anything that you are not ready to address yet?

_____

_____

_____

_____

_____

_____

What change do you want to make?

_____

_____

_____

_____

_____

_____

What scares you most about this change?

_____

_____

_____

_____

_____

_____

What excites you the most about making this change?

_____

_____

_____

_____

_____

_____

What obstacles might get in your way?

_____

_____

_____

_____

How can you overcome these obstacles?

_____

_____

_____

_____

Obstacles aren't impediments. Don't let them convince you to stop. View them as challenges—learning opportunities. The Universe tests the strength of your resolve as you strive for a goal. Obstacles provide a reason to flex your muscles and dig deeper than you thought you could.

We must hold tightly to our goals—our dreams—our aspirations—and yearn for them to the point we can taste, smell and see them. In our inevitable moments of self-doubt, we have a choice. We can allow the negativity to drown us in the sea of unknowing, or we can use our strengths—our bravery—to turn that self-doubt into a raft that will carry us to our destination.

The sea of unknowing—our self-doubt—wants to drown us. It is one of the culprits behind the development of disease. However, the way we think about our situation is just as powerful, if not more so, than the problem itself.

The mind is mighty. I've had clients who convinced themselves that autoimmunity lurked just around the corner. Some believed they had it already. They remained sure despite labs proving otherwise. I like to call this "Borrowing Trouble." We get so convinced that something will happen that we somehow think it into existence. Sure enough, those same clients within one year developed an autoimmune condition despite taking every precaution they could.

Conversely, I've also had clients come to me previously diagnosed with an autoimmune condition. They consumed an anti-inflammatory diet, exercised, drank adequate water, took quality supplements, etc., and yet did not see any abatement in their symptoms. My coaches and I work specifically with these clients on addressing their underlying emotional and mental strongholds. Typically, we see a high level of self-doubt and a low level of self-worth. As self-doubt declines, self-worth increases. The symptoms abate with this restored balance, and the client begins to feel better. How we think about ourselves and our situations makes a tremendous impact on our ability to heal.

I had worked with Maria for over a year when she started getting frustrated with her progress. With a previous diagnosis of Hypothyroidism and Hashimoto's, her Rheumatologist expressed concern that other autoimmune conditions lurked on the horizon. Wanting to avoid pharmaceuticals, Maria came to me to look for holes in her diet that might be contributing to her symptoms and the progression of her conditions.

We looked at her hormones, gut function, and food sensitivities, then used what we learned to co-create a plan to help her feel better. She followed everything to the letter. She eased up on her exercise, permitting herself to participate in gentler exercises. She adhered to her diet plan. She slept. Yet, she reported at each session that her energy levels remained low, and her symptoms persisted.

We adjusted various things, including foods, timing of nutrition, length of sleep, amount of water, etc. You name it, and we tried it! I finally looked at my emotional and frustrated client and asked, "Maria, do you think you are worthy of healing?"

She replied, "No, not really. I mean, I try, but there is just so much wrong with me." And with that, the tears streamed down her face. We found the root cause. She looked up at me and asked if that explained her lack of improvement. I nodded and said, "It's entirely possible."

After making this realization, Maria made efforts to change her thought patterns. She felt heard, and she knew she had a safe space to work through her negative emotions and build her sense of self-worth. The act of listening to her inner self allowed her to see symptom abatement finally.

*   *   *

We don't yet know the extent of how powerfully our thoughts affect the neurological system. But we do know that how we see ourselves determines who we are. What we think—we become. What we expect to happen—happens. Therefore, what we want—we can achieve. Our neurological systems don't differentiate between positive and negative thought patterns. Negativity is just as powerful, if not more so, as positivity. Whichever side you feed is the side that grows strong. (Remember the two wolves?) It will either drag you down or build you up. Either way—you choose!

This next activity is often the most challenging. Here, I ask you to be vulnerable with yourself and face the thoughts you have about who you are and what you look like. You will be naked for this next activity so make sure you have some privacy. Find a quiet place with a mirror. Remove your clothing, take a couple of deep cleansing breaths, and stand in front of the mirror. What do you see? What are your eyes drawn to first?

_____

_____

_____

_____

_____

_____

How do you feel about what you see?

_____

_____

_____

_____

_____

_____

_____

_____

_____

_____

_____

_____

Where do those thoughts come from? Are they your story or a story given to you? Be careful to consider, here, the story given to you by the media as well, especially if those thoughts are critical ones.

_____

_____

_____

_____

_____

_____

What do you like about your body?

_____

_____

_____

_____

_____

_____

Was it challenging to find something you like? If so, why?

_____

_____

_____

_____

_____

_____

_____

_____

_____

_____

Spend 10 minutes each morning or night repeating this activity for one week. Try to notice a different positive feature about your body each time. This activity may feel challenging at first, but it should get easier as time progresses. Reflect on your experience—either in a journal or in contemplative thought. Remember to return to these positive thoughts when you catch yourself falling, returning to negative thought patterns.

What is one thought pattern that you want to release?

_____

_____

_____

_____

_____

_____

_____

_____

_____

_____

When trying to reverse old thought patterns, have at least one person in your inner circle with whom you can share your struggles and joys. Who is that person for you? Why did you choose him/her/them? (Think about their qualities that you admire.) Do you have more than one person?

_____

_____

_____

_____

_____

_____

Section 5: The Immune System

1. In defense of it all
2. Cold or Emotional Exhaustion?
3. The Dis-ease Debate
4. Infection of Unhappiness and the Lack of Sweetness

We live in a society that values *doing* over *being*. When did you last lie around and do nothing conventionally productive? Did you watch movies? Read a book cover-to-cover? Did you feel guilty for taking that time? Most of us hear that nagging voice reminding us of everything we need to do. Sometimes we stay busy as a way of avoidance. We believe we can "beat" our anxiety if we just keep busy. We distract ourselves from the real issues. As time progresses, we exhaust our minds and bodies. We find it harder to think, and the quality of our work declines. Even more devastating, our quality of life deteriorates. Yet, we still feel compelled to push through because we're rewarded for that work ethic.

Instead of putting ourselves first, we repeatedly prioritize the greater good of the company, the community, or the family. We spend so much time making sure that everyone has what they need and that they are happy. By the time we fulfill our external commitments, we are left with scraps of time, if any at all.

What if we didn't do that anymore? What if we prioritized ourselves and said "no" to other commitments? What might we gain? At first, we'll struggle to silence our guilty sense of obligation. However, as we continually practice this skill, we will find it easier to prioritize ourselves without nagging voices questioning our worth when we don't say yes. When we quiet our inner judge, our inner child can come out to play.

The first step toward achieving this is simply to recognize. We can start to remedy the situation if we first identify it. When we cut a finger, we recognize the injury and put a bandage on it. We can't address what we don't take the time to see.

Why is it, then, that we don't take time to heal when we get sick (mentally, emotionally, or physically)? For some people, their financial situation dictates that they take as little time as possible off from work. Others might have too many people relying on us to take time off. And still, others may feel the overwhelming guilt of not living up to some arbitrary standards.

What is your greatest struggle with taking time for yourself?

_____

_____

_____

_____

_____

What things prevent you from doing the activities you enjoy?

_____

_____

_____

_____

_____

_____

_____

_____

Which of those things could you reduce because they're nonessential?

_____

_____

_____

_____

_____

Adding things to our to-do lists increases our stress load, so let's quickly review how our bodies respond. The adrenal glands produce cortisol, allowing us to enter the fight-or-flight state. This quick burst helped save our lives back in caveman time, but with today's constant stressors, we can struggle to release the stress response. The adrenals create a gateway of sorts to other systems, as well. The longer we maintain this state, the more our bodies must pull from stored resources. We've already examined the effect stress has on the small intestine.

Since the adrenals also keep the immune system well-oiled, stress can inhibit efficient immune responses, affecting the gastrointestinal, endocrine (hormones), and neurological systems. You can see the chain reaction stress causes throughout the body. The immune system impacts just about every other system, either directly or indirectly. The current medical paradigm continually attempts to isolate the immune system—an impossible task, at best!

For now, let's focus our attention on the connection between the immune and gastrointestinal systems, starting with the small intestine. Stress depletes the overall number of enterocytes—the intestinal tract cells—which weakens the intestines.

Think about the last time you were stressed out. How did your stomach feel? Did your body respond with nausea? Cramping? Diarrhea? Constipation? Did you feel like eating a lot or not at all?

_____

_____

_____

_____

_____

_____

_____

_____

_____

Our bodies have their unique ways of physically responding to our everyday emotional stresses. Take note of how your body responds so you can honor what it asks of you. When we slow down enough to listen to our bodies, we can slow down the deterioration occurring at a cellular level.

When we ignore our bodies and continue to push the stress down and move forward, the intestinal tract suffers. As the enterocytes struggle to reproduce, the gut lining struggles to keep the outside world (our food) from the inside world (the bloodstream). This affects the immune system, partly located in the small intestine. This is the junction where food allergies and sensitivities develop. If this barrage continues, the immune system cannot differentiate between toxin and self (or body).

The result of this constant barrage is autoimmunity, where the immune system no longer possesses the ability to distinguish intruder from self. Those who have experienced an autoimmunity diagnosis know how devastating it can be and how little reassurance accompanies it. Typically, the patient tries a prescription, and when that one fails, adds another one—and then another . . . and another . . . and another. . . Each medication carries side effects, eventually leaving the patient no better off than before. In many cases, the patient ends up in worse condition.

While this is normal in our current medical paradigm, it doesn't have to be the answer. We don't have a deficiency of drugs. We have damaged immune systems that need repair. A diet change may help to remediate missing nutrients, which is often a root cause of disease.

*   *   *

Gut-Immune Connection

At least once every 5-7 years, I catch a cold. I don't like being sick, and I do everything I can to avoid it, but eventually, I encounter a germ while my body's defenses are down. Typically, I am a head cold woman. My symptoms tend to localize with a stuffy and runny nose, headache, and all the other glorious and sexy cold symptoms. As an entrepreneur, a mom, a perpetual student, and a professor, I find myself saying, "suck it up" when I should listen to my body's demands and rest. I push myself to the point of exhaustion, as do many other women out there. I work with women holding 2-3 jobs just to make ends meet. Others try to keep it all together while their marital lives fall apart. Some put in overtime to build a career from two strings and a few pennies because that's all they have left.

On top of all of that stress, it is easy to eat foods that cause gut health imbalance. One of the most common things that I reach for when I am stressed is carbohydrates. I love me some muffins! Sadly, they don't feel the same way about me! This is very common. Carbohydrates trigger the production of serotonin, a chemical that produces feelings of well-being and happiness, in the gut. It's no wonder that we want comfort foods often high in starch and carbs when we aren't feeling quite like ourselves. Instead of addressing the emotions, we stuff them and our stress down into our guts hidden beneath layers of sugar and breads!

I get it! Ladies, I get it! We try to have it all and be it all, but we're exhausting ourselves at the price of our health. How much more impactful would our time spent on tasks or with our loved ones be if we took time for ourselves—sick or well—instead of putting ourselves last? Maybe if we did this consistently, we would be less likely to get sick. We could take time off to be well, instead.

* * *

Two theories exist—the germ theory and the terrain theory. The Germ Theory, credited to Louis Pasteur, Joseph Lister, and Robert Koch, states that the germ causes sickness. We happen to encounter the germ, and illness ensues. This theory does not account for the times we encounter the germ but don't fall ill. We encounter germs all day long, so shouldn't we be sick all the time?

The Terrain Theory, credited to Claude Bernard, states that the germ can take hold when our body provides a hospitable host. How does our terrain become hospitable? It does so through a lack of quality sleep, quality nutrition, and exercise.

Though highly summarized, these descriptions should give you enough of a picture to help you decide which theory supports your body and at which time. Both ideas are relevant and are intertwined when we look at a person's overall health and well-being. As we learn to address the stressors in our lives, we can fully support and enhance our immune system by providing extra nutrients—not just calories. We must create a terrain that is not welcoming to the germs that are all around us.

On his deathbed, Louis Pasteur purportedly said, "Bernard was correct. I was wrong. The microbe [germ] is nothing. The terrain [milieu] is everything."

In reality, both theories are valid. Our bodies fight germs regularly and are ever-vigilant to fight them. However, when smoking, drugs, alcohol, poor quality diet, lack of exercise or sleep, and high levels of stress damages the terrain, it has a much harder time trying to fight.

I recently had a client tell me of her daily stressors. Initially, she was a high-paid executive, but she and her husband decided she would stay home to raise their two children. She intended to return to her career when the youngest turned two, but at that time, she found out she had Lyme Disease. This illness, with new symptoms, always manifesting, leaves an individual feeling weak, hopeless, and completely debilitated. My client faced a long, frustrating fight to regain her health.

She shared her desires to be heard, regain her original health, and feel more in control of her life. In our first coaching session, she shared that she felt fear more than anything daily. She feared she would never again feel good health. She feared she would never be fully present and alive for her two children. She repeatedly asked me through her tears when she would be able to breathe again. My heart ached for her.

Naturally, I give my clients an assignment to focus on until our next appointment. She had enough on her plate, and adding one more thing would have likely been counterproductive. So, I kept hers simple, asking that she focus on breathing.

Over the next few weeks, we started breaking apart her fear.

* * *

What images does the word *disease* call to mind? Does the word invoke fear? Does it inspire you to make changes or look for new solutions? Earlier, we discussed the concept of disease. Feel free to review if needed.

Happiness is not a matter of intensity but of balance and order and rhythm and harmony.

—Thomas Merton

To bring back balance, the physical systems must be considered individually *and* as a functioning unit altogether. This is where conventional medicine often missteps in treating conditions.

When my son was younger, he liked to meticulously set out brilliant blue railroad tracks across my living room floor. They wound around the furniture (and dogs), under the tables, and up the single step that led to the rest of the house. At 3-years-old, my son envisioned his ideal track, and he would build it.

It didn't always work out correctly. Sometimes, the wrong ends of two tracks met up, so they didn't fit. Other times, the pieces fit, but the trains drove around the same loop repeatedly because the track had a "block" in it.

The same thing can happen in our bodies, which can leave us in a state of *dis-ease*. If we don't have the right building blocks (think macronutrients of protein, fats, and carbs here) combined with the proper levels of micronutrients (vitamins and minerals), the tracks fail to connect correctly. Or if we have all of the right pieces physically, but we have an emotional block on our track, we will spin in the same circles over and over, trying to figure out what we need to change before we burn out from exhaustion.

Let's return to my son's railroad tracks. I loved to sit and watch while he played with them. Since my son was independent from the moment he shot out of the uterus, I had to sit where he couldn't see me. As I listened in on his conversations with himself, I learned how his brain processed things. He is a lot like me—very logical and analytical in most of his interactions. That is, until the trains left the track. Whether due to speed differences or one of our cats playing Cat-Zilla, when those trains flew off the track, my son's thought processes moved from his head to his heart, and his emotions took over. He shed tears and threw a fit until he was ready to put the train and track right.

Sometimes we have to take those moments. We have to feel and express our emotions in healthy ways. Once we've processed them, we can let them go and return to our task at hand— whether it's an emotional conflict, a change in our physical status, or any other situation that might throw us off-kilter. There is nothing we can't handle, and we are so much stronger than we give ourselves credit for.

Think of something that has changed for you. How do you see this contributing to your overall health status? What does this situation bring to your life?

_____

_____

_____

_____

_____

_____

_____

_____

_____

What can you do to change your current situation?

_____

_____

_____

_____

_____

_____

_____

_____

What emotions do you have surrounding your current situation?

_____

_____

_____

_____

_____

How do you see these emotions impacting your health?

_____

_____

_____

_____

_____

_____

_____

_____

Have you sat with your emotions? If you have, what was that like? If you haven't, what is stopping you from doing so?

_____

_____

_____

_____

_____

_____

_____

_____

_____

_____

You may not be able to change your current situation, but you *can* change how you react to or feel about it. I remember seeing a poster in my high school counselor's office. It said,

> *I am convinced that life is 10% what happens to me and 90% how I react to it. And so, it is with you . . . we are in charge of our attitudes.*

—Charles Swindoll

At that moment, I realized that I could control how I responded to a situation, even if I couldn't control the situation. We don't have the superpower to control everything that happens to us, but we have the superpower to control our reactions.

What can you do to change the way you are feeling?

_____

_____

_____

_____

_____

_____

_____

_____

_____

_____

How could changing your emotions (or reaction) to the current
situation help your overall physical health?

_____

_____

_____

_____

_____

_____

_____

Your emotions guide you and help you to understand your fellow humans, but through generations of conditioning, many of us have learned to stuff our feelings. They represent the "girlie" side of our human existence and thus require hiding. A great divide has existed between masculine and feminine for too long, even though they both exist within each of us. Fortunately, we as a society have slowed the drive toward exclusive masculinity and begun the turn toward a kinder, gentler balance of our innate masculine and feminine energies.

I mentioned in an earlier chapter that your tribe is important—critical, even—to make the changes you desire. As you change your thinking patterns, you may notice that you question the people with whom you associate. Misery still loves company. For example, what fuels the water-cooler conversation at work? Most likely, it's the negative stuff. So-and-so got laid off, and did you see what so-and-so is eating/driving/wearing? When we pass judgment on someone, we bring more people down to that level. Walk away from it. Maybe one day, you will even feel confident enough to confront it. Remember, if you aren't part of the solution, you are part of the problem.

You either have to be part of the solution, or you're going to be part of the problem.

—T. Siedner, London NW2

Finding the Sweetness in Your Life

One of the things we tend to reach for when we're sad is sugar. This temporary lift in our spirits results from a short burst of serotonin production. You feel good, and you want more . . . more sugar, that is! Sugar is eight times more addictive than crack, and it lights up the same opioid sensors in the brain. No wonder we crave more.

Our bodies are hard-wired to want to find sources of sugar and fat because they are our bodies' two significant sources of energy. Our Paleolithic ancestors survived by bingeing on it when they found it, but they also had long periods without it. Mind you, they weren't drinking sodas and eating baked goods. Their sugar came from fruits.

We modern humans don't have those long periods of famine. We can run to the convenience store, grab something sweet, and return to our sedentary job under fluorescent lights. While not everyone is in this situation, a large portion of our society is. We have changed the way we live in the name of progress. Yet, one thing is clear. We've removed the sweetness of life in the name of progress. We work more hours and spend fewer hours with the ones that we love. We abandon hobbies or interests because there isn't enough time in the day after our 8 to 10-hour shift and 1-3 hours of commuting time. We're barely lucky to shove food in our faces, fall asleep in front of the television and start the process over again tomorrow.

We explored in a previous chapter the idea of returning to fun and of rekindling those hobbies and interests. Now may be a great time to review that assignment and make sure that you are still on track with it. If you fell off the wagon, make sure you climb back on and make some time for those things. I know that there has been a movement in our culture for work/life balance, but what if we had *life*/work balance where our lives came first? How much happier might you be? How much more quality time could you spend with those you love? Where can you find the sweetness in your own life right at this moment?

This lack of sweetness drives us to grab the foods we innately and intuitively know that our bodies don't want.

Is your sweet-craving tainted?

Here in the United States (and many other countries), our sweetness comes with a hefty dose of genetically modified organisms. Our addiction to sugary emptiness is killing us in a lot of ways. The rise of Insulin Resistance, Metabolic Syndrome, Type 2 Diabetes, Alzheimer's Disease—all driven by imbalances of sugar—is also driven by an increased amount of genetically modified organisms (think high fructose corn syrup) and a decreased amount of pleasure/fun in our lives.

Since the early 1980s, our food supply has been genetically modified to supposedly create higher crop yields driven by the fear that our food supply would be insufficient to meet the demands of our ever-burgeoning society. The issue with GMO crops is that they are combining protein structures that don't naturally occur in nature, and our bodies don't know what to do with them. Many of the crops contain pesticides/herbicides already built into them to help deter crop damage. While this book is not about GMO's, I think it's worth mentioning because they affect our gut health. If you are looking for a more in-depth conversation about genetically modified foods and what they do to our health, I would highly recommend checking out *Genetic Roulette: The Gamble of our Lives* by Jeffery Smith, which won the movie of the year by the Solari Report in 2012.

What health or personal conditions would you like to see change?

_____

_____

_____

_____

_____

What are you willing to do to get to where you want to be?

_____

_____

_____

_____

_____

_____

_____

_____

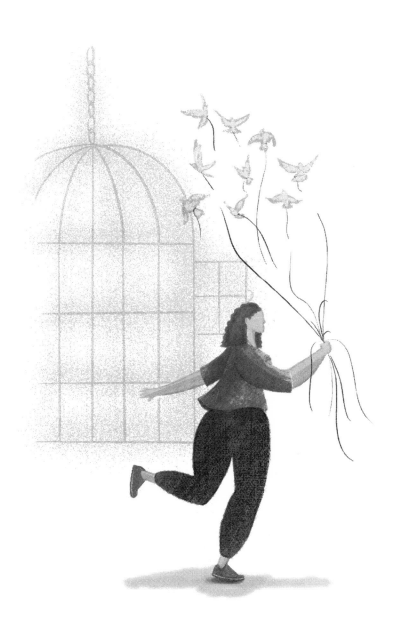

CHAPTER 6

It's Your Turn

And So, She Decided to Live the Life She Had Always Dreamed

Each person's journey to healing starts at a different point, but every journey begins with the first step. You've taken your first step by working through this book. Applaud yourself! You could have picked up any other book today, but you chose this one. Every step—no matter how small or large—deserves celebration. Your next step is to decide how to move forward.

What are you willing to do to get to where you want to be? What things or people are you now ready to give up or to add to your life to build your health?

_____

_____

_____

_____

_____

_____

_____

_____

_____

Now that you have identified the things that you are still facing, the only thing left to do is to figure out what to put in your "suitcase." You examined your strengths and maybe found ones that you didn't realize you had along the way. You brought your goals, desires, and interests into focus. You played captain of your team and chose who would join you on your journey because, after all, no woman is an island. *You* did all of this, dear reader. You have more strength in your heart than you ever thought you had.

What are some of the obstacles that you think you might encounter along your journey from this point forward, and how will you address them? What do you have in your "suitcase" to help you?

_____

_____

_____

_____

_____

_____

_____

_____

_____

_____

_____

_____

It only takes one small step to get you moving away from your old self to move toward your new self. This is the symbolic death of the old self. You can manifest your future by getting comfortable in the place of the unknown—otherwise, you are just living the same patterns over and over. You aren't living at all.

You can't hold on to the past and step into the future entirely. Search the internet for motivational speeches. There is no shortage of influential speakers and videos to help you get on your way. Just remember that motivation comes from within. Look for reminders all around you. Allow your friends, family, nature, co-workers, or random strangers to cheer you on and support you. Opening up and allowing yourself to be vulnerable is scary—at times downright terrifying—but you have accomplished so much in such a short period. When you feel like everything is too much all at once, allow yourself the space to return to the safety of your heart and home. Regroup. Identify and befriend emotions, and then be prepared to let them go when they no longer serve you.

Changes never truly last if you make them for someone or something else. You have to do this for yourself, but know that you have a support system behind you. Over the last few pages, you have identified the people who love and support you. You have identified those people who you allow to hold you back. You have taken the time to celebrate your victories, and you have set new goals for yourself.

Remember, sometimes we encounter smaller victories that give us signs of more significant accomplishments down the road. For example, if you want to purchase a home this year, don't overlook the new apartment. It's a little cheaper and gets you away from your crazy neighbors!

You may want to return to an earlier exercise and consider revising it. One of my favorites to revise is my narrative, that exercise where you identified the truths and lies about who you are. Now that you have completed the book and the activities in it, this may be a great time to rewrite your story and then compare the two. I would be willing to bet that they changed.

On average, it takes six full weeks to adopt a new way of thinking or behaving. Give yourself a break! Change is tough. Trust me, I know. Change keeps me awake at night and leaves me feeling uneasy until it's over, no matter how beneficial I know that change will be. If it takes you a little longer than others to make your desired changes, that is ok. There is no competition—no race—here.

This is **your** journey to healing your body and bringing wholeness to your world. It does not matter what other readers are doing. It does not matter what others in your circle or tribe are doing. This moment is about you. It is about what you want to achieve and who you want to become.

It is time to run toward those things that will help you accomplish your desires. Ask yourself, who am I? What do I want? Where do I see myself in 3, 5, 10 years? What do I need to do to make this happen? Notice that each of these questions uses the pronoun "I." Whatever others say or think about you is no longer your business. Your business is your happiness and joy. Let go of expectations based on stories you have been given and write your own.

Self-Care, Selfishness, Self-Centeredness?

There is a massive distinction between being selfish and being self-centered. Early on, I talked about balance and learning to say no. It's never an easy thing for us women to remember. We have been taught to say yes. In those times that you feel like you are wavering in your commitment to yourself, return to the feelings of being able to say no without the guilt and meditate on them. This time focusing on yourself is not time wasted, Dear One. It is a reminder of your worth. I often ask my clients to be selfish but not self-centered. Selfish means you put yourself first and to do the things that make you happy. This happiness makes you more fun to be around and more likely to accomplish the things you want. It makes you a better spouse, lover, friend, dog-walker, etc. Who else will put you first—truly first—without any self-serving motives? Only you can do this for yourself, Dear One.

Being self-centered means that you think the world revolves around you and your shit doesn't stink. Quite frankly, everyone's does, so let's just get over this one and move on. Everyone's world doesn't revolve around you—just your own.

Dear One, in this final exercise, I want you to write two letters to yourself. The first letter will be your current self writing a letter to your future self. The second letter will be your future self writing a letter to your present self. What do you want to say to yourselves?

Letter to your current self from your future self:

_____

_____

_____

_____

_____

_____

_____

_____

_____

_____

_____

_____

_____

_____

_____

_____

_____

_____

_____

_____

_____

_____

_____

_____

_____

Letter from your future self to your current self:

_____

_____

_____

_____

_____

_____

_____

_____

_____

_____

_____

_____

_____

_____

_____

_____

Staying in the positive light and energy won't always be easy, but the more time you spend there, the more the Universe will hear and respond to your desires.

You are worth putting first. You are worth empowerment and forgiveness. You deserve the time and effort required to focus on the things you want. I leave you with this final thought:

If we were meant to live mediocre lives, why are there so many brilliant people doing extraordinary things every day? (Psst, Dear One, you are meant to be one of them.)

With Love and Light,
Dr. Jennifer Champion

Note to the Reader

*P*lease take a moment to provide a review of my book. I would love to hear what this book has done for you.

As a special bonus, I have a free gift for you to get you headed in the right direction nutritionally and to build personal resilience. Nutrition is a frontline defense in helping you build your confidence and maintain your strength, emotionally and physically. Go to http://www.neogenesisnutrition.com/journey_to_wholeness/ to sign up for my mailing list. By joining, you will receive monthly articles and information about upcoming events on living the life you want with success, health, and happiness.

About the Author

Dr. Jennifer Champion DCN, MS, CNS, FMCHC, CN, is a Board Certified Clinical Nutritionist, Health Coach, Author, Educator, Speaker and Owner of NeoGenesis Nutrition, Inc., an Integrative Nutrition practice based out of the greater Tacoma area. She 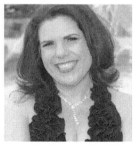 believes in the idea of empowerment when it comes to addressing health concerns. Too many times, patients are told what to do, but are never consulted along the way. Education is power when it comes to making an informed choice about your current health goals.

Dr. Champion addresses the underlying causes of your symptoms in a bottom-up approach instead of a top-down approach that is our current medical paradigm. The symptoms are warning signs, but not the cause. At 20 years-old, Dr. Champion realized that she needed to make some changes to save her own life. Being offered only prescriptions and no real advice on how to make changes in her life that would support her desire for optimal health, she set out to figure out how to help herself. Having weighed 350 pounds and been diagnosed with PCOS, depression, anxiety, and infertility, she knew that there had to be connections between what she was eating and how she was living that was contributing to the development of her dis-ease. This ignited a passion for helping others figure out the puzzles to their health.

Dr. Jennifer Champion holds a Masters in Human Nutrition and Functional Medicine from the University of Western States in Portland, Oregon and a Doctorate in Clinical Nutrition from Maryland University of Integrative Health. For more about Dr. Jennifer Champion or to work with her, please visit her website at www.NeoGenesisNutrition.com.

Made in the USA
Middletown, DE
31 March 2021